Crack Your Code

The Ultimate DIY Guide For a Thinner, Happier Life

Chris Barlics

The ideas, procedures and information contained in this book are intended for information
purposes only and are not intended as a substitute for consulting your physician or healthcare
provider. All matters regarding your health require medical supervision. This book is not meant
to be used, nor should it be used, to diagnose or treat any medical condition. For diagnosis or
treatment of any medical problem, consult your own physician. The publisher and author are
not responsible for any specific health or allergy needs that may require medical supervision and
are not liable for any damages or negative consequences from any treatment, action, application
or preparation, to any person reading or following the information in this book.

For my mom, Diane.

Contents

Introduction

"The combination of your WHY and HOWs is as exclusively yours as your fingerprint." -Simon Sinek

I never thought of my mom as overweight. She was just my mom. To others she was also a nursery-school teacher, an active member of the PTA, a former catechist of the year, a devoted daughter who cared for her aging parents, a loyal friend, and a loving wife. She left an indelible positive mark on the lives of so many. Yet a lot of her self-esteem and self-worth were predicated on only one thing—her weight.

Once, when I was in seventh grade, I tried to play hooky from school because I was being bullied. My mom sat down on my bed and had a heart-to-heart discussion with me, sharing with me that she too used to be bullied. Kids used to pick on her for being "fat," she explained, which made her hate school and look down on herself.

Weight loss became a lifelong journey for my mom. Willing to try anything, she joined walking groups, did countless diets, took aerobics classes, followed along with Richard Simmons tapes, and purchased a treadmill for our basement. I even remember a cartoon image of the character "ALF" pinned to a corkboard on our refrigerator. ALF sat next to an overstuffed picnic basket, underneath the saying, "Those who indulge, bulge." It was a gentle reminder for her not to overindulge.

When it came to the weight-loss industry, my mom was a perpetual consumer, always buying, yet never fully attaining her desired result. She tried every fad, only to watch the results she achieved vanish easier than they came. Unfortunately, my mom's lack of results robbed her of much more than her self-esteem.

In 2004, my mom was diagnosed with breast cancer. Soon after completing chemo and radiation, she went into remission, and we all thought she was in the clear. Then one Sunday in March of 2009, she went to the ER and discovered it had come back—and that it had metastasized to her brain in the form of dozens of inoperable tumors. Three short months later, at the age of only 54, she passed away. Just like that, she was gone.

Thinking about all the things my mom wanted to do but never got the chance to do breaks my heart. She never traveled to Italy. She never realized her dream of owning a beach house. Saddest of all, as much as she loved kids, she never got to meet her own grandson. It often leaves me pondering the what-ifs.

What if my mom had figured out years earlier how to live a healthier lifestyle? Would it have mattered? What if she stopped following all the fad diets and exercise gimmicks and found a path that actually got her results? How much better would her time on Earth have been? Most importantly, would she still be with us today, enjoying time with her grandson?

My mom took care of everyone—except herself. I often wish she had made her health more of a priority, especially since studies now show that being overweight increases the risk of breast cancer for postmenopausal women by up to 60 percent.

I'm sharing this with you because it's been ten years and I'm still angry—but not at my mom. I'm angry at the weight-loss industry that failed her. I blame their greed and the convoluted, deceptive way they "encourage" their customers.

The weight-loss industry wants perpetual consumers. Many within it care a lot about making money and very little about getting people—like my mom—sustainable results. The magical products or "scientifically proven systems" they sell are nothing but smoke and mirrors designed to make us hope and hand over our money, while, in the end, what we end up losing with these programs are our money and hope. We are left wondering if lasting weight loss is even possible.

Since you're reading this book, I'm guessing that you don't feel like you are where you want to be when it comes to health and fitness. Perhaps you too have tried diets you eventually gave up on or exercise programs you started and stopped more times than you care to count. Maybe you bought expensive equipment, joined a gym, or even hired a trainer. Some of it probably worked for a little while, but I bet some of it didn't work at all.

Whether you identify your goal as losing weight, getting thinner, losing fat, getting toned, etc., you are here looking for answers—answers that are probably connected to some difficult questions, such as, how do you make the necessary changes when changing feels so hard—especially in this crazy, stressful world?

How do you change your eating habits when food may be one of the few things that gives you pleasure and a sense of comfort? How are you supposed to exercise consistently when you're exhausted and there doesn't seem to be enough time in the day—and when doing so causes you discomfort?

My goal is to help you find the answers to these tough questions and many more. But before we talk about those, I want to address the one question I'm asked more than any other: *How do I lose weight once and for all?* After all, this question is probably what brought you here.

The difficult thing is that when most people ask this question, they are looking for a magical formula to follow that will help them lose weight quickly and easily. Maybe you have tried the typical "eat less and exercise more" strategies and discovered that you're able to sustain them for only so only long … and that eventually they lead you right back where you began.

If this happened to you, I bet you thought you were the problem—that you were weak, unmotivated, or lacked willpower. The truth is that you are not the problem, your strategy is.

We've been taught to listen to the so-called experts and influencers who arrogantly think they know what's best for us. If you ask a dozen different experts how to lose weight, you'll probably get a dozen different answers. In the end, though, they are all cookie-cutter strategies that fail to take into account the most important variable: we are all unique.

Each of us has our own individual characteristics that make us who we are. We live in different places, and we have different lifestyles, schedules, histories, quirks, needs, values, preferences, DNA, etc. While many of these may seem similar to other people, there are nuances within each characteristic that, when combined, make up a profile that is unique to only us.

The path to achieving your goals is out there, but it isn't in some prepackaged program or step-by-step system. It is composed of a unique set of strategies that takes into account all your unique variables. You just need to know how to find it! I think of it like cracking your own personal weight-loss code. Right now, that code is a mystery; but it's one that can be solved.

Throughout my fifteen-year career, I have helped hundreds of clients lose weight. I have studied the science around weight loss and continue to spend numerous hours dissecting the latest research. Despite all of this, I have no idea what combination of strategies will work for you. If they're being honest, neither does any other health or fitness expert. Only one person can figure out how to solve this mystery that lies before you, and that's you! This is your mystery, and that makes you the lead detective!

Think of this book as detective's school—a practical guide, one that gets straight to the point without a lot of fluff. It will help you identify the issues that need solving and give you a blueprint for solving them in a way that works for you. Each chapter in this book discusses a different weight-loss variable—everything from mindset, habits, and willpower to practical tips for nutrition and exercise, to motivation and behavior change—and how to apply them to the context of your life.

Together, we will discuss many proven weight-loss concepts and strategies, but my hope is you'll view these as a menu of options from which to pick, rather than a step-by-step system. Essentially, I'm giving you a bunch of puzzle pieces and teaching you how to sort through them to figure out which ones you need and how they best fit together to create the outcome you desire. Rather than trying to mold yourself to fit a game plan someone else gave you, I will teach you how to develop a game plan that works for you and your life.

I'm hoping the pages that follow provide you with a different perspective about what you're trying to accomplish and that this book empowers you to get off the crazy train of fads, gimmicks, and bad science. I never had the chance to help my mom, but if she were still here and asked me for help, the conversation would probably look something like this:

Mom: *"Chris, how do I lose weight?"*

Me: *"You need to understand the basics of how weight loss works and then follow them using strategies that work for you."*

Mom: *"Okay, but how do I do that?"*

Me: *"Read this book. I will show you how."*

I would like to believe this book would have helped her, just like I hope it helps you. If you're ready to stop bouncing around from method to method and begin learning how to crack your specific weight-loss code once and for all, then you've come to the right place!

PART 1: THE WHY

Chapter 1

A Billion Dollar Mystery

"Whenever you find yourself on the side of the majority, it's time to pause and reflect." -Mark Twain

S ome things in life should probably remain a mystery: the origins of the universe, who really shot JFK, and what animal parts are really used in hot dogs. Some things we're just better off not knowing—but how to lose weight and feel your best are not among them. The truth is, though, losing weight is more confusing than it has ever been. Each day adds more to the ever-growing amount of contradictory information that keeps us stuck and unsure what to believe or where to start.

For thousands of years and using many different methods, people have tried losing weight for many different reasons. Historically, it seems to have all started with the ancient Greeks. In fact, if you're ever on Jeopardy, the word diet comes from the Greek word *diatia*, meaning a lifelong regimen for health. To the ancient Greeks, having a healthy diet and engaging in regular physical activity ensured a healthy society; thus, it was the civic duty of all citizens.

Much later in America and Europe, between the fifth and 16th centuries, being overweight held the opposite connotation. It was associated with affluence and success, as only the wealthy could afford to overindulge. However, over the next few hundred years, being overweight regained its negative stigma.

The Victorian era of the 1800s was an age of prosperity and peace for England, but it was the age of stupidity for health. Many risked their well-being in search of a slimmer waist. People wore corsets to mold their abdomens, took diet pills even though they were known to contain arsenic, and even came up with the brilliant "tapeworm diet," ingesting tapeworms to lose weight.

As time went on, people became a bit smarter about their weight-loss strategies, but things continued to get worse. Industrialization and scientific advances increased food availability, which meant that weight gain became an issue for everyone, not just the wealthy. As more people attempted to lose weight, more weight-loss strategies appeared.

"The cigarette diet," which was lead by the Lucky Strike cigarette company, emerged in 1925 with the slogan, "Reach for a Lucky instead of a sweet." Diet pills made a comeback, this time using amphetamines as the main ingredient, which had very serious, life-threatening consequences.

During the Great Depression, people took a break from caring about losing weight as most people were just trying to survive. However, after it was over and food was overabundant once again, many new weight-loss strategies emerged. The grapefruit diet, which required people to have a grapefruit before every meal to help them lose weight, became popular. And Weight Watchers, created by New York housewife Jean Nidetch, was born in 1961.

By the 1970s, the weight-loss industry was booming, and fad diets were the craze. SlimFast and Lean Cuisine both launched. Extremely restrictive diets such as the "cabbage soup diet" emerged, but it mainly just gave people gas. During the late '70s to early '80s, fat became the most demonized macronutrient, which changed in the '90s, when carbohydrates became the enemy and the Atkins and Paleo diets grew in popularity. Then everyone was scared of trans fats (rightfully so) until sugar recently became the villain.

Despite Jack LaLanne's 1960s syndicated television show, most people still just focused on dieting. The exercise craze didn't really enter the mix until the 1980s, when exercise gadgets and fads (not to mention the tight, shiny, neon workout clothing) were also being sold. That's when Jane Fonda, who is largely credited with popularizing fitness for women with her VHS tapes, came on the scene. Richard Simmons immediately followed, along with many others.

Slowly, as the volume of products and strategies on the market grew, so did consumer confusion. Today, things are more confusing than ever before. With so much contradictory information, nobody knows what to believe.

When Oprah recently became a major shareholder in Weight Watchers, she bragged about losing weight while still eating bread. But the South Beach Diet talks about limiting white bread, white rice, white pasta, baked goods, alcohol, and fruit—which is contradicted by the Mediterranean diet, which says fruits, along with vegetables and healthy fats, are fine.

Many systems like Weight Watchers talk about counting Calories or "points." However, the Whole 30 program tells consumers to forget about Calories and just focus on eating natural foods.

Now, since the popularity of the ketogenic diet has soared, it seems we're back to demonizing carbs and sugar. Others are starting to realize that prepackaged diets aren't the answer and are eating based on their genetics—a field of study called nutrigenomics. With so many possibilities, it's hard to know who to believe or where to start, isn't it?

To add to the confusion, many claim you can eat whatever you want as long as you burn it off through exercise, which is why the Bowflex, Total Gym, Tae Bo, P90X, Wii Fit, Sauna Suits, Power Wristbands, Shake Weight, Beach Body, and the Ab Lounge—just to name a few—have had their fifteen minutes of fame.

If this weren't enough to make your head spin, there are dozens of other approaches to weight loss, from the more "passive" methods such as the pyramid-scheming diet plans Isagenix and Herbalife, to the meal-delivery systems such as Nutrisystem. Intermittent fasting has even made a comeback, not to mention hypnosis and other "mindset" training systems. There are also countless weight-loss apps, including My-FitnessPal and Noom.

The Mystery Remains

One would think, with all of these different programs and resources at our disposal, that achieving and maintaining a healthy weight would be much easier than it was a hundred years ago. However, data reveals that it's getting even harder. Obesity rates have more than tripled since the

1950s. It is estimated that over 70 percent of US adults are now overweight or obese. And it's not from lack of trying.

According to a report from the National Center for Health Statistics, 49 percent of American adults try to lose weight each year, and those who try fail 97 percent of the time. Many who initially lose it regain most of it within six months.

It seems the more weight-loss products and plans that emerge, the more weight we gain. Looking back at the history of the weight-loss industry, we see that virtually every angle has been covered: low carb, low fat, low sugar, high protein, "eat just whole foods," Calorie-counting, point-counting, "don't count anything just drink shakes," move more often, don't eat for 12 hours, home-delivered meals, ingest tapeworms, etc.

All of these strategies help the weight-loss industry rake in over $70 billion annually, yet as individuals and as a society, sustainable weight loss is still a mystery. It begs the question, is losing weight and keeping it off even possible?

Proof That It Is Possible

In 1994 Dr. Rena Wing and Dr. James Hill launched what has become one of the largest weight-loss research groups in the world. The National Weight Control Registry is a study that examines the strategies of over 10,000 members who have each lost an average of 66 pounds and have kept it off for an average of six years and counting.

On the surface, the findings seem unremarkable. Ninety-eight percent of participants reported modifying their food intake in order to lose weight. Ninety-four percent increased their physical activity. Seems obvious, right? But what is important to note is that this is where the similarities end. The only other thing all 10,000 participants have in common is that they each found a way that worked for them.

This proves three things. First, many people have been successful at losing weight. If they can succeed, so can you. Second, contrary to what marketers tell you, there is no one best system or path to losing weight. And third, the key to lasting weight-loss success is to find a path that works for you. That is what each of these 10,000 participants did, and that is what this book will teach you how to do.

Your Unique Weight Loss Code

We've gotten so used to looking to external sources for answers that it becomes hard to imagine any other option. With all the books, blogs, new articles, and videos on the Internet, we think the answer must surely be somewhere! There are and will always be a lot of people—doctors, personal trainers, dietitians, annoying friends—telling you what they think you "should do" to lose weight. Different diets, exercise systems, meal plans, supplements, and step-by-step programs—everyone will tell you something different.

"You should stop eating carbs."
"You should do an hour of cardio per day."
"You should do intermittent fasting."
"Do these types of exercises!"

Almost everything invented in the last hundred years has a "Trust me, I know what will work for you better than you do" vibe about it.

Yes, somewhere within all of this contradictory information are valuable strategies and key concepts that will help you hit your goals. However, I can promise you that your keys do not lie in someone else's prepackaged, step-by-step system or quick-fix fad. Instead, your keys lie within an iterative process of self-discovery, where you piece together little strategies to form a unique system that works just for you. This mysterious system is what I refer to as your Weight Loss Code.

Becoming A Weight-Loss Detective

Many who struggle with losing weight have what I call the "passenger's mindset." They treat their goal as if they were calling an Uber. They choose their destination and want someone else to figure out the route, while they exert as little effort as possible. This may be an efficient way to get around, but it has been proven ineffective for long-term weight loss. To be successful, you simply cannot be a passenger on your own journey!

As of now, NOBODY has figured out what works for you—perhaps because nobody else has the clues to crack your weight-loss code but you.

It's time to come to terms with the fact that cracking this elusive code is a job only you can do. The majority of those who sustainably change how they look, feel, and live are the ones who have what I call a "detective's mindset." They don't follow "done for you" programs. They don't search for easy answers on Google. They are very much "DIY," creating their own program from a unique combination of strategies, tools, and resources.

At the end of the day, your success is not determined by what anyone else says or thinks; it is determined 100 percent by what you do. During a time when most are following flashy, perfectly packaged programs promising quick and easy results, it's time to consider taking a different route. While a path focused on cracking your code can sound mundane, as you'll soon find out, it is the only path that can guarantee success!

Your weight-loss code is out there, waiting for you to crack it. It's time to get out of the backseat and get behind the wheel on a journey to self-discovery. Once you stop letting other voices drown out your own, you'll be able to find strategies that work for you, in your life, for your goals. Everything you need to crack your weight-loss code is already inside you. Now it's time to bring it to the surface!

Key Points

- Despite the ever-growing amount of tools and resources that have come out over the last few hundred years, weight loss remains a mystery for millions.

- The world's largest weight loss study comprised of over 10,000 people reveals that there are three keys to losing weight: modifying food intake, increasing physical activity, and finding a way to do both that works for you.

- Experts will pretend to know what will work for you so you will buy their product.

- Your path to success doesn't lie in passively following someone else's "prepackaged" diet or exercise program, it lies with you becoming more self-aware and figuring out what will work for you.

- Those who struggle do so because of their "passenger's mindset." Those who are successful have a "detective's mindset."

- Your path to success will be made up of a number of particular strategies combined in a way to work for your lifestyle, your preferences and your goals. This is known as your weight loss code.

- Despite past frustrations, rest assured that your code IS out there. But nobody is going to discover it for you. Only you can! Throughout this book, we will explore everything you need to know to crack this code

Chapter 2

The Battle For Your Mindset

"Love yourself first, then everything else falls in line." -Lucille Ball

"Your self-worth is determined by you. You don't have to depend on someone telling you who you are." -Beyoncé

I t sounds a bit like a conspiracy theory, but the last thing that the weight-loss industry wants you to do is to come up with a plan to crack your code. Why? Because if you successfully lose weight, you'll no longer be a customer. They profit when you're lost, unhappy, and always buying the next best product or plan.

Everyone has an angle. The media only cares about you paying attention to their stories. Authors only care about you buying books. Doctors get bonuses when you take medication. Health and fitness celebrities just want you to follow them. And fitness and nutrition entrepreneurs want you to buy their products or supplements.

Marketers spend millions and millions of dollars each year trying to convince us that we're broken. Their goal is to make us feel so bad about ourselves that we collectively spend billions and billions of dollars on products and services that promise to "fix" our flaws.

For instance, many chain gyms measure a personal trainer's success by how many clients they sell, not by how many clients they help achieve goals. I once knew a trainer who was known as the "sales guru" of his company. He would often brag that his method for acquiring clients was to make a person feel so bad about how they looked that they'd be willing to pay anything to fix it. His motto was, "If you make them cry, they'll buy."

Unfortunately, as you'll see, many in the weight-loss industry share this attitude. They care a lot about making money, not about helping you reach your goals, and they are ready to take advantage of any vulnerability. So before we talk about how to crack your code, let's discuss the dirty tactics they use to convince you to keep following them, so you'll be able to recognize them and become immune to their games.

Smoke, Mirrors And Photoshop

Marketers have crammed "thin equals popular" and "popular equals happy" down our throats. Everywhere we look—in magazines and on television and our social media feeds—we are surrounded by "gods and goddesses." The constant, subtle message, "If you want to be popular and happy, you need to look like this" is unavoidable, but internalizing this message can do serious damage to our self-esteem. It can cause us to think, "Well, I don't look like that but I wish I did, so what do I have to do to get there?"

They want us to internalize the message because then they hit us with the sales pitch. We've all seen an ad displaying a toned model next to a headline that reads "Get Abs like These in Only 5 Minutes a Day," but the reality is that you won't look like the model doing only five minutes a day. The model didn't even get those abs by using that program. Like many other fitness models and trainers I know, they got paid to endorse a product or system they have never used. Secondly, chances are the model doesn't even look the way they do in that picture! Many times that picture is the result of a descent physique enhanced by lighting, camera angles, and photoshop.

Marketers use these methods because they work like a charm. After all, smiley, airbrushed models promoting a flashy system that promises simple, easy success can be hard to resist. We spend our hard-earned money hoping these products will help us, and when they don't, our self-esteem plummets even more and we start doubting our ability to lose weight.

Awareness Equals Power

Before and after pictures are another tactic marketers use to "prove" that their product works. While this seems logical, these photos are often misleading. In 2013, an Australia-based trainer named Mel V took her own transformative before and after bikini pictures of herself. When she shared them, many wondered what great diet and/or exercise program she was using, but the truth was she didn't use any program at all. Both pictures were taken only fifteen minutes apart!

While it certainly looked like she followed a special 90-day program, all she did was use the marketers' tricks—she played with angles, lighting, and her wardrobe. For the "before" picture, she stood close to the camera, wore red bikini bottoms that were a bit small, put her hair up, and slouched, relaxing her stomach. For the "after" picture, she gave herself a quick spray tan, stood farther away from the camera, wore black bikini bottoms that were larger, let her hair down, changed her posture, and tightened her stomach.

It is really easy for a fit person to change their posture and stick out their stomach. It is even easier for a photographer to photoshop a model until they look flawless. Although these "tricks" may seem trivial, the damage they can cause is not. They create a false ideal that is impossible to reach. They can persuade us (and our younger generation) to measure our self-worth only by how we look and how much we weigh. And they can lead us down the wrong path to quick fixes and bogus strategies that set us farther back from actually achieving our health and fitness goals.

These pictures, infomercials, and social media posts do not depict real life. They exist only to get us to spend money. What gives us—the consumer—power is being aware of the game that these marketers play so that we can start becoming immune.

Good Things Take Time

Nobody has ever said, "I want results, but I wish I had to work super hard for a long, long time to get them." We humans are always looking for the most efficient way to do anything, a trait that marketers exploit by intentionally making us feel broken and then promising us fast results with their cleanses, pills, and exercise gadgets.

Even though society is getting better at spotting BS, a lot of fads still gain momentum because those who use them often initially lose weight. When they do, others take notice and want to know how that person lost weight. Before long, word of mouth starts to spread that this product or system "really works." Voila, a fad is born.

Unfortunately, the issue becomes short-term vs. sustainable results. After the excitement of a fad wears off, so do the results. Before long, everyone ends up back where they started because the methods used in these quick fixes are about as sustainable as putting duct tape on a broken pipe. Sure, it might temporarily appear to work, but when your kitchen floor gets soaked after washing the dishes, you realize that it wasn't such a great idea after all.

Despite hearing this, many will continue looking for quick, easy solutions to a problem that requires a lot of time and investigation to solve. They keep believing that the next program will be "the one" and that this time will be different, except it never is.

The Quick Fix Irony

The search for a quick fix is actually quite ironic. Many spend decades looking for the shortest, fastest way to weight loss, yet after twenty years, they're no closer to achieving their goal. If you're looking only to lose weight fast, it will take you an eternity to be successful. All of these quick-fix illusions blind us to the process that actually works.

If you believe that fit, healthy people achieved their results using a crash diet or an infomercial fitness product, then you've already lost. Those who are successful do not buy into fads. They become investigators who use self-awareness and a lot of trial and error.

We All Have Blooper Reels

When pursuing a goal, it can be really discouraging to look around and constantly see people farther along than we are or people making faster progress. I often hear people say how frustrating it is that their spouse or friend lost weight so quickly, yet it's taking them much longer, or that their spouse can eat everything in sight and not gain any weight.

While on the surface this may not seem fair, focusing on what others are doing only hinders your progress. Every ounce of mental energy spent looking at someone else takes the focus off what matters most—your own journey.

If you are going to learn something from others' success, consider this: the success you see in others is merely the tip of the iceberg. There's so much more under the surface. Everyone struggles, and everyone feels like quitting. The tip of the iceberg does not allow us to see all the frustration, sacrifice, doubt, fear, discomfort, and failures they experienced along the way. Take social media, for example. Everyone on social media posts flattering pictures of themselves, but how many other unflattering pictures did they take before getting the good one?

If you feel like you often get discouraged when comparing yourself to others, remember that everyone overcame their own struggle—and you need to overcome yours. The only person you're competing with is yourself. As long as you stay focused on moving in the right direction (even if you're moving slowly), you WILL reach your goal!

Support Yourself

I know this sounds a little strange, but we talk to ourselves each and every day - maybe not out loud (although I definitely do from time to time), but through our thoughts. Every time we think, we're speaking inwardly. It's like our own private conversation, yet because it's so automatic, we seldom notice what we're saying to ourselves.

Think about it: how do you usually speak to yourself? Are you polite and encouraging or rude and insulting? If most of us spoke to other people the way we often speak to ourselves, nobody would want to be around us. In fact, our self-talk could probably be considered verbally abusive at times. Our doubts, fears, and insecurities enter our head, and we begin to drown ourselves in mean, discouraging words without realizing the harmful impact they can have.

Whether you're willing to accept it or not, this negative self-talk is affecting how you feel about yourself, and it is limiting your ability to reach your goals. This is something with which everybody struggles.

So then why do we do this to ourselves, and how can we stop? I'm not sure there's an easy answer to that question. One explanation is that we're all inner perfectionists. We demand a lot from ourselves, and we think that if we aren't hard enough on ourselves, we will never do what is necessary to achieve our goals.

Whenever we fail to do something, it's easy to fall into the trap of thinking we need to be stricter or harder on ourselves. On the surface, this makes sense because when we're young, our brain's self-control system isn't fully developed, so we learn self-control through our parents' commands and punishment. Unfortunately, many of us still talk to ourselves like abusive parents. This typically doesn't work.

Trying to "light a fire under our rears" will only eventually burn us. Initially it might make us feel motivated, but this lasts for only a short while. Studies have shown that self-criticism diminishes self-esteem, robs us of motivation, and makes it harder to have self-control. In the end, it leads to us seeking out ways to comfort ourselves—hello, Netflix and comfort food!

If you feel you would like to improve in this area, consider practicing more self-compassion. Catch yourself when you start speaking to yourself harshly, and instead, act like you were talking with someone you loved and respected. I realize this is much easier said than done, but the first step is to listen to yourself. Awareness is always essential when making a change.

Just to be clear, I'm not suggesting that you be loosey-goosey with yourself and let whatever happens happen. That's not a recipe for success either. What I am advocating is that you challenge yourself, but when you stumble, encourage yourself instead of beating yourself up. Accept that stumbling is an essential part of the process. Treat each stumble as experience from which to learn. Ask yourself, "What lessons can I take away from this that will make me better on my next try?"

Bottom line, be careful how you talk to yourself because you are listening! It will be much easier to crack your code and create sustainable change if you treat yourself with love.

You Are Worth It!

Contrary to what marketers want you to believe, you, my friend, are not broken! The answer to your mystery does not lie with a new piece of exercise equipment or the next greatest diet to hit the market. It lies primarily within you!

Everything in this book becomes a lot easier when you really start believing in yourself and the power you have. You will want to exercise more, eat better, and take care of yourself. You will want to put the pieces together—not because you want to impress someone else or look like the airbrushed models you see on social media, but because you will realize what I already know without ever having met you: you deserve to be healthy and happy!

Key Points

- The weight loss industry doesn't want us to be successful because finding our own path to losing weight will save us thousands and cost the weight loss industry billions.

- Marketers spend millions of dollars using tactics to manipulate us into feeling broken so we will go out and spend money buying their "quick fixes."

- Continuing to search for quick fixes will only take us further away from reaching our long-term goals.

- The only person we're competing with on our journey is ourselves - focusing on the progress of others will only distract us, frustrate us and take energy away from making key discoveries.

- Listen to how you talk to yourself - focusing on creating more positive self-talk, especially during the tough times, will help keep yourself motivated and moving forward.

- The more you believe in yourself and shut out all of the distractions around you, the more likely you will be to crack your code.

Chapter 3

You Are Much More Than A Number On A Scale

"Start with Why." -Simon Sinek

We give the scale a lot of power, don't we? We let it dictate everything from our mood to how we feel about ourselves. If we lose weight, we feel happy and hopeful. If we don't—or worse, if we gain weight—we feel defeated.

It is important to reflect on the fact that the scale measures only one thing— our relationship with gravity. It doesn't measure how kind we are, how valuable we are, or how much good we do or potential we have. We are all so much more than a number on a scale or the inches around our waist. Too often, we let a number negate our greatness. We may be excellent parents, loving spouses, loyal and supportive friends, caring people, skilled professionals, and/or valued members of our community. No scale in the world can quantify these qualities, yet they truly matter!

Does this mean that weight loss shouldn't be a priority and that you should learn to be happy with where you are and not strive to better yourself? Only you can answer that. This process is not about what I want you to do, nor is it about what your doctor wants you to do. It's not about what your friends or family want you to do. It's only about what YOU (and you alone) want to do.

I wrote this book for people who are frustrated and feel stuck with their fitness and health goals and want to change. If you're happy with where you are and don't intend to change, that's awesome! Maybe you've decided that life is too short, that you would rather continue eating the way you normally do, and that you get enough physical activity already. I'm not trying to convince you that you need to change anything. Nobody should!

However, if you are unhappy with where you are; if you really want to feel better, be healthier, and look better, you can either keep making excuses for why you haven't gotten it done, or you can start making it happen! This does not mean you're admitting that you don't like yourself—quite the contrary. It means you love yourself so much that you are willing to do what it takes to take care of yourself and be the best possible version of you.

Too many people view weight loss from the perspective that either you should strive to lose weight, or you should learn to value yourself and learn body acceptance. It doesn't have to be so binary. Realizing that you are awesome just the way you are is the most important goal to achieve. But trying to be the healthiest, strongest, fittest version of yourself is equally as awesome.

I hope that your happiness doesn't hinge on you losing weight, but I also hope that you realize you are worth taking care of—that this journey is worth seeing through, no matter how many twists and turns there are along the way.

The path to weight-loss success is often long and winding, which is why it helps to have a guiding light. Before we start discussing the details of how to start putting the puzzle pieces together, it helps to know what we want the final picture to look like. Let's first define exactly WHY you want to embark on this journey.

What Does Success Look Like For You?

"What's your goal?" Whenever I ask clients this question, the answer typically starts with, "I want to lose X number of pounds." After asking a few more questions, though, it becomes obvious that their goal is so much deeper. The number on the scale is just a superficial representation of what they are actually trying to achieve—similar to winning the lottery. Nobody wants to win just because they want large sums of money sitting in their bank account. People want to win the lottery because of how the money will make them feel and what it will allow them to do or to buy.

Success with fitness and health means something different to everyone. It could mean fitting into skinny jeans, attracting a mate, or being able to get off blood-pressure medication. It could mean being accepted by others, being around for your children and grandchildren, or being able to walk up the stairs without being out of breath. Everybody's version of success is different.

Frederic Nietzsche once said that those with a strong WHY can bear almost any how. Losing weight is not easy. It requires a lot of patience, mental energy, strategizing, learning, sacrifice, and consistency over a long period of time. On a journey riddled with obstacles, traffic jams, and detours, it is essential to remind yourself of WHY you want to crack your weight-loss code.

Autonomy is essential. Your goal isn't about making others happy. It's not about what anyone is telling you that you should do. It's solely about what success means for you. What does your version of success look like?

If you're having some trouble connecting with your why, start by asking yourself the following questions:

> *What does success look like for me?*
>
> *If I were successful, what would that mean for me and those around me?*
>
> *How would I know if I were successful?*
>
> *How will it change my life for the better?*
>
> *What could happen if I do nothing different and keep doing what I'm cur-rently   doing?*

Cultivating Your Vision

Once you have a strong grasp on your WHY, consider turning it into a vision statement: one or two sentences detailing how you would like to feel, who you would like to be, and how you would like to live your life.

While creating a vision statement isn't essential, it can be quite helpful. Like we discussed, it is not uncommon to find ourselves becoming so obsessed with the number on the scale that we lose sight of our real motivators. Creating a vision statement requires you to concisely verbalize your goals and helps you paint a clear picture that provides you with both inspiration and direction, especially when you feel discouraged.

To craft your vision statement, start by thinking about the following questions:

What do I want my life to look like in one year? In five, 10, and 30 years?

What personal values are important to me? (For example, independence, fun, family, career success, contributing to society, autonomy, happiness, peace of mind, self-respect, and achievement)

What would my ideal day look like?

To get the ideas flowing, here are vision statements that a few of my clients have created in the past:

Example Vision #1: *I want to set a great example for my children and to feel physically strong and energetic so that I can thrive and handle life's demands. I want to feel vigorous and youthful, making physical activity part of my everyday life.*

Example Vision #2: *I want to feel young and vibrant so that I can travel through life with confidence, energy, and vigor. I want to feel physically capable and ready to take on whatever challenges life throws my way.*

Example Vision #3: *I want to be a fit, healthy, independent grandmother who is able to play with my grandkids and has full freedom to enjoy life.*

My clients have found it helpful to keep a copy of their vision statement in places like the kitchen, their car, and their office. Some even turned it into a graphic on their cell phone or laptop. The key is to put it somewhere that your "future self" is likely to see it when you need some extra motivation.

A Mystery Worth Solving

The code you're trying to crack is not just about hitting a number on a scale or fitting into your skinny jeans. It probably is connected with you feeling happier and living longer. A 2017 study found that being overweight or obese was responsible for more preventable deaths in the US than smoking. If achieving your goal meant having more time here on Earth doing the things you love with the ones you love, what could possibly be worth more? But what I say doesn't matter—you need to believe that cracking your code is worth your time.

Once you have a strong sense of your vision, the next step is to start figuring out how to make it a reality. After all, a vision without an actionable plan is nothing more than a dream. Constantly obsessing about the outcome does nothing to get us closer to achieving it—which is why you need to figure out a path that will work for you.

Key Points

- The scale does not measure your worth, it just measures your relationship with gravity. You are so much more than how much you weigh!

- Cracking your code is about so much more than pounds, body fat or inches. It's about your health, your happiness, and everything that's important for you.

- Everyone has their own personal reasons for losing weight. Dig deep inside yourself and find your WHY.

- Once you know your WHY, create a vision statement and strategically place it in locations where you will see it. It can serve as a reminder of what's important to you when you are in need of motivation.

PART 2: THE FUNDAMENTALS

How To Crack Your Code

Chapter 4

The Facts Of Weight Loss

"It is a capital mistake to theorize in advance of the facts. Insensibly one begins to twist facts to suit theories, instead of theories to suit facts." -Sherlock Holmes

One of the big tragedies within the world of weight loss is how misunderstood the physiological mechanisms of losing weight really are. People overcomplicate the simple stuff and oversimplify the stuff that requires a lot of attention.

Although the path that will lead to your weight-loss goal might still be a mystery, the good news is that the mechanism for losing weight is not. Weight loss occurs as a result of an energy deficit in the body. In other words, when we consistently burn more Calories than we consume, we lose weight.

Lately, there are those who say that this answer is too simple. While it is true that many factors influence how many Calories we expend and how many we eat, that doesn't change the fact that weight loss happens only when there is an energy deficit in the body. Some think that this is wrong because, in their mind, they've done that and it didn't work. As we'll see, many of us overestimate the number of Calories we're burning and greatly underestimate the number of Calories we're consuming.

If you have gained weight, then more days than not, you've consumed more Calories than you've burned. If your weight is not changing, then you're eating and burning the same number of Calories. The focus remains Calories in vs. Calories out.

While this formula may seem simple, within it are many complexities that are essential to understand. Getting to the bottom of this formula will help you better identify clues, come up with new strategies, and help you connect different pieces of the puzzle that may have been missing. But you must have a firm grasp of the facts. Let us first take a step back and start from the beginning.

What Exactly Is A Calorie?

A Calorie, (note the uppercase C) also known as a kcal, is a unit of heat measurement. Technically speaking, it represents the amount of heat necessary to raise the temperature of one kilogram of water by one degree Celsius. In case you're curious, a calorie, spelled with a lowercase C, is a small calorie representing the amount of heat needed to raise the temperature of one gram of water by one degree Celsius. When we think of food, we almost always think in terms of kcals or Calories.

A Calorie is a unit of energy containing about four joules, which is why people use the phrases "energy deficit" and "Calorie deficit" interchangeably. Calories are calculated by placing food in a bomb calorimeter—a sealed container surrounded by water. The food is then completely burned, and the rise in water temperature is measured; this gives us the number of Calories in that particular food.

While knowing what a Calorie is and how it's calculated might be great, the big question everyone asks is, "How many Calories can I eat if I want to lose weight?" The answer is almost entirely dependent on how much energy you expend per day. Therefore, before you can determine how many Calories you can eat per day, you first must figure out how many Calories you burn each day.

Calculating Caloric Output

When most people think of burning Calories, they think of exercise. Surprisingly, though, physical activity is just a small part of total Caloric expenditure - accounting for only 15-30 percent. We also burn Calories through two other sources. Here's the complete formula:

Total Caloric Expenditure = Basal Metabolic Rate + Activity + Thermic Effect of Food

If we want to accurately measure how many Calories we burn, we need to know how to calculate expenditure from each of these three sources. Let's start with the biggest one.

Basal Metabolic Rate

Of all the Calories burned throughout the day, 50–70 percent come from our basal metabolic rate, known by many as our "metabolism." Simply put, our BMR is a measure of how much energy our body uses at rest.

Trying to estimate how many Calories you need to consume to lose weight without knowing your BMR would be as effective as creating a budget without knowing how much money you earn. So how do you calculate it? There are several formulas you can use. Here are the two most popular:

Mifflin-St. Jeor Equation

Men: (10 x weight in kg) + (6.25 x height in centimeters) - (5 x age in years)

Women: (10 x weight in kg) + (6.25 x height in centimeters) - (4.92 x age in years)

Katch-McArdle Equation (using lean body mass)

Men & Women: 370 + (21.6 x lean body mass in kg)

When calculating, keep in mind the following:

1 inch = 2.54 centimeters

1 kg = 2.2 lbs

If you hate math as much as me, your eyes probably hurt just looking at these formulas, but stay with me. Let's try an example together. Let's say Kathy is 47 years old, stands five feet four inches tall (162.56 cm), weighs 162 pounds (73.63 kg), and has 34 percent body fat (48.6 kg lean body mass). Calculating her BMR would go as follows:

With the Mifflin-St. Jeor equation:

(10 x 73.63) + (6.25 x 162.56) - (4.92 x 47)

736.3 + 1,160 - 231.24 = 1,521.06

With the Katch-McArdle equation:

370 + (21.6 x 48.6)

370 + 1,049.76 = 1,419.76

As you can see, these formulas will give you slightly different answers. The Mifflin-St Jeor formula incorporates your age, while the Katch-McArdle takes into account your lean body mass. So which one should you use? Rather than choosing one (since they are estimations anyway), I recommend you start by calculating both formulas and then averaging the two answers. This would mean Kathy's average BMR would be roughly 1,471 kcal per day.

One thing to note is that, while the Mifflin-St Jeor calculation can be done with the information you have right now, you first need to have your lean body mass (aka body fat) measured to use the Katch-McArdle equation. This is an extra step, but it's worth doing. Body composition significantly impacts our metabolic rate. Many gyms offer body-fat measurements at little to no extra charge.

Thermic Effect Of Feeding

Did you know we also burn Calories when we digest food? It's called our thermic effect of food (TEF). In total, it accounts for around 10 percent of our daily Caloric expenditure.

The general rule for estimating your TEF is to take the total number of Calories you eat per day and multiply it by 10 percent. For example, if you ate 1,600 Calories today, your TEF would be approximately 160 Calories. It's important to note that this is just an estimation. Your number could be higher or lower, depending on the types of foods you eat. We'll cover this in Chapter Seven.

Physical Activity

The most widely considered form of energy expenditure is physical activity, which is broken down into two categories: Calories we burn from exercise and Calories we burn from everyday activities, also known as NEAT (non-exercise activity thermogenesis).

Even calculating how many Calories we burn from physical activity isn't as simple as you might think. Many factors influence it, such as age (typically the older you are, the fewer Calories you burn), body size (metabolism is typically a bit higher the more you weigh), and gender (males usually burn more Calories than females).

A simple way to calculate your total Caloric expenditure from physical activity would be to wear a Calorie tracker, like a Fitbit. While many get sick of wearing one after several months, it is a good tool to gain awareness. Another way is to guesstimate it by multiplying your BMR (that you calculated earlier) by the number that best describes your activity level below:

1.2 = Sedentary lifestyle (desk job, little to no formal exercise)

1.3–1.4 = Light activity and light exercise 1–3 days per week

1.5–1.6 = Moderate daily activity and moderate exercise 3–5 days per week

1.7–1.8 = Very active lifestyle and hard exercise 6–7 days per week

1.9–2.2 = Athlete in endurance training and/or a very physically demanding job

Using 47-year-old Kathy, who has an average BMR of 1,470.41 and walks approximately three days a week while engaging in light activity throughout the day, her formula would be as follows:

1,470.41 x 1.4 = 2,058.57 Calories expended from BMR + physical activity. Factor in that she typically eats 1,600 Calories per day, making her thermic effect of food about 160, then her total Caloric expenditure would be as follows:

1,470.41 + 588.16 + 160 = 2,218.57

In sum, Caloric expenditure = BMR + physical activity(NEAT + Exercise) + TEF. Once you figure your estimated Caloric expenditure total, you will have the information you need to come up with your average daily Caloric intake goal.

Calculating Caloric Intake

Once you've calculated your average daily Calorie expenditure, you can now focus on the "Calories in" portion of the formula. So, back to that million-dollar question: exactly how many Calories can you eat and still lose weight? The trick lies in creating a deficit that's big enough to get results but not so big that you're starving and damaging your metabolism. This is where you really need that detective's hat!

It has long been believed that averaging a 500 Calorie per-day deficit will yield a weight loss of one pound per week. A while back, researchers found that a pound of body fat contained approximately 3,500 Calories. So they concluded that if someone wants to lose a pound of fat per week, they need to eat 500 fewer Calories per day than they expend (3500/7= 500).

The problem with this is that not everybody loses weight in a linear fashion. Many factors determine how much of a Caloric deficit will result in noticeable weight loss. Current body weight and body-fat percentage both need to be taken into account. For example, if someone weighs 270 pounds and has a higher amount of body fat, they will tend to drop weight a lot quicker than someone who weighs 170 pounds and has less body fat. Another factor is that as you lose weight, your metabolism will lower because fueling someone weighing 270 pounds requires more energy than someone who is 170 pounds.

So, while a 500-Calorie deficit might be a good place to start your investigation, I recommend experimenting with a deficit range of between 10 and 25 percent. For most people, this means eating between 200 and 600 fewer Calories than you expend.

How do you know where in this range you should fall? Testing is better than guessing! See how you feel. Make sure you're getting an adequate balance of protein, fiber, carbs, and healthy fats. And—spoiler alert—the more whole foods you eat, the higher your TEF will be and the fuller you'll feel.

Tracking Your Calorie Intake

Can you lose weight without tracking Calories? Absolutely! Remember, the only thing determining right from wrong is if it makes sense as a long-term option for you. However, I do have a word of caution: it will be much harder to analyze and make the necessary initial adjustments if you don't first track your Calories for at least a little while.

Without tracking, many people underestimate how many Calories they consume. A study in the UK found that people consume up to 50 percent more Calories than they think they do. Collecting data from 4,000 people over four days, they found that women reported consuming an average of 1,570 Calories per day but actually consumed an average of 2,393. Men reported consuming an average of 2,065 but actually consumed 3,119.

If you are going to be able to identify changes that need to be made, you need to know where you currently are. We balance our checkbooks so that we don't overdraw our bank accounts. If we don't track Calories, many of us will go over our Calorie targets and gain weight. Good detectives leave no stone unturned. While it isn't always ideal to do long-term, I strongly recommend tracking Calories at least for the first few weeks to gain awareness. Remember, you don't always have to count Calories, but Calories always count!

With regards to tracking Calories, there are several different methods from which to choose. The most objective method is to use a food scale and measuring cups to measure food quantities. Once you know how much of each food you eat, you can go online and research Calories. Then it's just a matter of recording and totaling them up in a food diary or a nutrition app. My clients have had success using apps such as MyFitnessPal.

Another option, which I refer to as the "hand method," is easier but not nearly as accurate. You eyeball serving sizes of food to see the appropriate portion size. One of the most popular ways of doing this is to use your hand as a portion guide. Here's how:

For whole grains and starches, one serving equals about half a fist.

For lean protein, one serving equals approximately the size of one palm.

For vegetables and fruits, one serving equals approximately one fist (for leafy greens, two fistfuls is equal to one serving).

For healthy fats, one serving equals approximately one thumb length.

The third option, which has helped many, is to think about what you're currently eating and how you can make it a bit better. This option is especially great for those who have consistent, predictable eating habits. It will allow you to eat a bit less of what you currently eat or to make healthy substitutions. For example, if you typically have four slices of pizza, try cutting it to two or three. These small improvements can add up to big results.

Start with whichever option you feel will work for you. If you get good results, then keep doing what you're doing. If you don't, then be honest with yourself and try another option.

Not All Days Are Created Equal

You don't always have to eat the same amount of Calories each day - it's your weekly average that really matters. If you do decide to count your Calories, consider budgeting your Calories during the week according to your lifestyle. For instance, let's say that based on your expenditure, your average daily Calorie target is 1,800. This doesn't mean you have to limit yourself to 1,800 Calories every day of the week. Instead, you can use a strategy called Calorie cycling.

Calorie cycling means that if you normally eat out on Fridays and Saturdays and know your Calorie consumption will be higher on those days, you can adjust your Calorie targets accordingly. On Sunday through Thursday you may want to stick to eating 1,650 Calories per day so that on Friday and Saturday you can eat 2,200 Calories. At the end of the week, you still will have averaged 1,800 Calories per day.

Don't Make This Mistake

When Jessica began her fitness journey, she weighed 172 pounds, and her goal was to get to 149 pounds—her college weight. After four months of staying in a Calorie deficit thanks to consistent exercise and mindful eating, she lost a total of 18 pounds, only five pounds away from her goal.

But then her progress slowed, and eventually, the scale stopped moving. It would fluctuate a few pounds here and there, depending on water retention, but the average stayed the same. Jessica's mood and motivation completely sunk. She started feeling more tired, and her cravings dramatically increased.

Upset that her efforts were no longer paying off, she started displaying the "what difference does it make?" attitude. "Why am I putting myself through this if I'm not seeing any more results?" she thought. Frustration turned into anger, and anger turned into hopelessness. "Will it really make a difference if I skip the gym today?" she thought. "Why not have a second or third helping of pasta?" Slowly, the scale climbed back up, and before long, she was back to where she started. She blamed herself and her lack of self-control. Little did Jessica know, however, there might have been another cause.

Stories like Jessica's happen far too often. Regardless of whether something similar has happened to you in the past, I want you to be informed so that it doesn't happen to you in the future. The reason that Jessica and so many others fail to sustain their weight loss is that they're unknowingly violating a physiological concept called "the set point."

Our body prefers being in a state of homeostasis—the tendency of our bodies to resist change. What this means is that our body is happy where it is. If we drop too much weight too quickly, our body sees it as a threat and goes into survival mode, doing everything it can to try to get our weight back to where it was.

While this may not be noticeable at first, there are clues that our body is entering survival mode: Our appetite—especially for carbs— starts to increase. Our metabolism slows, making us feel tired and lethargic and preventing us from expending a lot of extra Calories. All of this persists until we return to our brain's comfortable set point.

Looking at things through this lens can give us another perspective on why keeping the weight off can be so hard. It's not because of a lack of willpower or motivation; it's because we're trying to lose too much weight too quickly. When we try to resist our body's natural survival mode, our brain will win—no matter how strong our will.

Consider following a method for losing weight that safely lowers your set point rather than resists it. Research shows that, on average, we should not aim to lose more than one to two pounds per week. More than that could trigger our body to go into survival mode. But that doesn't mean you should expect to lose this amount every week.

At first, you might lose three to four pounds and then the next week you'll lose one or two pounds. During the next two weeks you might not lose anything at all. For the weeks when the scale doesn't budge, don't panic. It doesn't mean your progress has stopped; it just means your body is recalibrating, which is a natural part of the process. Your body needs to take some time to adjust to the changes.

Everybody is different, but recalibration usually happens when you've lost about 10 percent of your original weight and it can take between four and 12 weeks. It's during this time that your body will create a new set point. This is when you will want to increase your intake so that it matches your expenditure (but not so much that you go into a surplus and start gaining weight). Once you adapt to a new set point, your body will no longer be fighting you and, after a few weeks, you can focus on creating a Caloric deficit to lose more weight (if desired).

While this might sound okay now, when you're in the middle of a plateau and the scale hasn't moved for several months, it is easy to get impatient. This is when most people throw in the towel. Remember, sustainable weight loss is created by understanding how your body works and working with it rather than against it. It may take a lot of patience, but slow, sustained weight loss is better than years of yo-yo dieting. A year from now, you'll thank yourself.

Finding Your Path

We've covered a lot of essential information in this chapter, but it alone probably won't provide you with the answers to crack your code. That's because these facts are worthless without action to make them happen.

Knowing about being in a Caloric deficit is one thing; figuring out how to do it consistently is something altogether different. Learning what methods and strategies to employ to make this happen for you requires great detective work. In the next chapter, we're going to discuss how to be a great detective.

Key Points

- Weight loss occurs when the amount of Calories you expend are greater than the amount of Calories you consume - also known as an energy deficit.

- The mystery lies in discovering how to maintain an energy deficit (and/or maintain an energy balance) so it is sustainable for you, in your life.

- To be successful, one needs a solid grasp of the fundamentals of Caloric expenditure and intake.

- Before you can figure out how many Calories you should eat, you need to first calculate how many you expend.

- Caloric Expenditure is more than just how many Calories you burn from exercise. It is the sum of three factors: Basal Metabolic rate, Physical Activity and Thermic Effect of Feeding.

- Once you have your Calorie intake goal, it is recommended that you track Calories, even if it's only for a few weeks to gain awareness.

- Using Calorie cycling can help you create a plan that accounts for your weekly activities.

- Losing too much weight too quickly causes our bodies to go into survival mode - making it nearly impossible to maintain. Understanding the Set Point Theory can help you plan a path that will make it easier to keep the weight off because you'll be working with your body instead of fighting against it.

Chapter 5

Becoming A Super Sleuth

"Stop looking for the answers from strangers. The answers to your life are within you. Only you know what makes your heart feel at home. Only you can hear your inner voice. The key is in asking the right questions." -C. Nordyke

Have you heard of Sir Arthur Conan Doyle? Most people haven't, but I bet you know his most famous creation—the character of Sherlock Holmes. In each book, Sherlock Holmes utilized powers of observation, analysis, and deduction to solve even the most impossible of mysteries. While the character may be fictitious, figuring out one's path to weight loss can seem just as impossible as a Sherlock Holmes case.

These days, most questions we have can be answered in seconds. When it comes to losing weight, however, the most important questions cannot be Googled - the ones that answer which strategies will work for you. This is your task! On this journey toward cracking your code, you are both the detective and the subject of investigation—which makes it especially challenging. But with the right mindset, learning how to ask the right questions, and having a system for finding the answers, you will be successful. The aim of this chapter is to provide you with these essential skills.

The Mindset Of A Detective

When working toward a goal, many envision the path to success as one straight line, a false expectation that causes many to quit prematurely. All it takes is one setback or a few bad days, and they throw in the towel.

Before we talk about methodology, let's first discuss one of the most important factors that will determine your success—your mindset. As you set out to crack your code, keep in mind that nobody gets it right the first time. True long-term change, the kind that sticks, is a continual process of taking three steps forward and two steps back.

One of the most important attributes you can possess during this process is patience—especially the patience to embrace failure, which is the necessary investment we need to make in order to be successful. Many view failure as time wasted. I disagree because if we learn something from the "missteps," then failure was not a waste. It becomes the most productive thing we could have done. Each failure provides us with new leads to investigate. The only real failure is not trying anything at all.

Cracking this code requires us to find the good clues within the bad days. It requires us to not fall into a "woe is me" mentality, and instead to put on our detective's hat, knowing the answer is out there. This means that, when we feel like nothing is working, we take a step back and ask ourselves, "What am I missing?"

Many call this process "trial and error." Since we're talking about having a detective's mindset, perhaps we should rename it "trial and learning."

Methodology

Best-selling author Josh Kaufman created a way to break down the process of trial and learning into an easy-to-follow framework. He calls it "the iteration cycle." While he created it for businesses, it can be applied to any venture—including weight loss. There are six steps to the cycle:

> Observe and Reflect
>
> Brainstorm
>
> Decide
>
> Implement
>
> Analyze
>
> Repeat

Step #1 – Observe And Reflect

Since you are both the detective and the subject in this journey, self-awareness is crucial. Becoming more self-aware starts by spending time focusing on your day-to-day habits, behaviors, and mindset. Doing so will provide you with the clues you'll need to start investigating further. Your task is to first identify two specific things: your change windows and your decision windows.

Identifying Your Change Windows

When people set out to lose weight, they often think they're solving a 24-hour problem. In reality, our results are dictated by a few behaviors we do or don't do during relatively small windows of time during the day.

To start cracking your code, look at your average day and figure out where your "danger windows" are. For example, when are you most likely to either consume excessive Calories or opt out of exercise? This is the window of time where you want to make a change—hence the name "change window."

Identifying Your Decision Windows

Okay, you've identified your change windows. That's awesome! The next step is to identify your decision windows, which are periods when you make the decision(s) that ultimately affect what you do during your change window. For instance, let's say your change window is between 10 and 11 p.m., when you would typically eat a whole pint of ice cream. To find your decision window, ask yourself, "When do I make the decision that sets me up for success or failure?" If you believe that you will eat the ice cream if it is in the house, then your decision window would be when you're at the grocery store. If you don't bring it into the house, you won't eat it.

You may still need to drill down a little deeper. For example, perhaps you buy the ice cream at the store because you go shopping when you're hungry. Therefore, maybe your decision window is the period of time right before you go to the store. If you ate something prior to shopping, you'd be less inclined to buy the ice cream.

This also works with fitting exercise into your life. As an example, suppose you've identified your change window and have a goal of going to the gym to work out for 30 minutes after dinner on Mondays at 7:30

p.m. And let's say that for the last few Mondays, despite your best intentions, you didn't make it. You need to figure out two things: First, what is your decision window? Second, what strategies might help you make a better decision? Here some questions that may help:

What would you like to have accomplished during that day (or that meal, or that period of time)?

What did you do instead?

How were you feeling (i.e. stressed, lonely, excited) when you engaged in the behavior in question?

Were you alone or with someone else?

What made engaging in this behavior possible?

What environment were you in?

As you answer these questions, you'll begin to see patterns emerge regarding how and why you make the decisions you do. To illustrate how this could work, here's a sample conversation I had recently with a client. We'll call him Sam:

Me: What would you like to have done on Monday night?
Sam: I would have liked to have made it to the gym after dinner.
Me: What did you do instead?

Sam: Stayed at home, did the dishes, and watched TV until bedtime.

Me: How were you feeling when you decided not to go to the gym?

Sam: I was exhausted from a long day.

Me: Were you alone or with someone else?

Sam: My wife was there.

Me: What made engaging in this behavior possible?

Sam: It was easy for me to use the excuse of being too tired to get up and go to the gym to work out. My wife agreed.

Me: What environment were you in when you made this decision?

Sam: I was home on the couch.

Once you've observed and reflected on the situation, then it's on to Step 2.

Step #2 – Brainstorm

After narrowing your "windows" and gaining some awareness, the next step is to brainstorm some strategies that might help you change your behavior(s). What options do you have for different choices? What could you change or improve? What skills do you have to learn? What might help you make a different decision next time? After spending some more time observing and reflecting (Step #1), I asked Sam to brainstorm some ideas. Here's what he came up with:

Me: What are some ideas you have that may help you make a different decision next time?

Sam: Instead of sitting on the couch right after dinner to rest, I could just leave for the gym right after dinner.

Me: How do you feel this option would benefit you?

Sam: For me, as soon as I sit on the couch, I know the chances of me getting back up to go out to the gym are slim to none.

Me: Are there other ideas you have or strategies you could use?

Sam: I suppose I could go straight to the gym after work, before I come home and eat dinner.

Me: How do you feel this option would benefit you?

Sam: It would eliminate any chance of me not going to the gym. I find that once I'm home, I get comfortable and start losing motivation to get to the gym. If I'm out driving already, I might be more likely to get to the gym.

Step #3 – Decide

Once you've brainstormed some strategies, it's time to decide for yourself which one makes the most sense to try first. Going back to the dialogue between Sam and me:

Me: Of the two strategies you've mentioned, which one would you would like to try first?

Sam: I think I'd like to try going to the gym right after work.

Me: Awesome. What, if anything, would you need to plan ahead of time to make this behavior possible?

Sam: The night before, I need to pack a gym bag with my workout clothes, water, and a towel and put the bag in my car so I can go straight from work to the gym without having to stop at home.

Me: Okay, let's make this strategy into a SMART goal ...

SMART Goals

When deciding what strategies to implement, it's important that we make them as clear as possible. Social scientist Al Switzler believes that a lack of desire or willpower can stem from a lack of clarity.

When trying to lose weight, many people simply say that they need to "eat better" or "exercise more." These aren't behavioral goals; they are just vague principles. Unfortunately, vague principles yield vague actions because they lack clarity and set us up for failure and frustration. As the saying goes, without a clear target, it's very difficult to aim.

One of the best ways to clarify our target is to make strategies that are SMART: **S**pecific, **M**easurable, **A**ctionable, **R**ealistic, and **T**ime-based. In case you are unfamiliar, let's review how you can ensure your strategy or goal is SMART.

The S stands for **specific**, which means that your goal should be as clear as possible. If it is unclear, you won't feel as motivated to accomplish it. To make sure your strategy is specific, think about answering the five W's—who, what, where, when, and why.

The M suggests that having **measurable** goals is crucial because it will enable you to track your progress. Assessing progress can help you stay focused, creating excitement as you get closer to achieving your goal. To make a goal measurable, think about the "how" questions: How will you know when you're successful? How much ...? How many ...? How often ...?

The A stands for **actionable**, meaning your goal should be based on a behavior, not an outcome. An actionable goal should be a behavior you can picture yourself doing, something specific and measurable that you could put on a calendar or a to-do list.

A common mistake people make when creating SMART goals is saying something like: *I'm going to lose 15 pounds in the next three months.* While this isn't necessarily wrong, it's an outcome goal; it isn't actionable. You will only find success if you identify the behaviors and strategies that will lead you to losing those 15 pounds.

Not only do you want your goal to be actionable, you also want to make sure it's **realistic**. Behavior-based goals are only useful if you do them. Ask yourself, is the behavior feasible? On a scale of 1–10, how confident do you feel that you'll be able to complete the task? If you're number is less than a nine or a 10, what might help you feel more confident about doing the task?

Finally, the T stands for **time-based**. Every goal needs a target date so that you are working toward a deadline. Making time-based goals helps prevent everyday tasks from taking priority over your goals. As famed author Stephen Covey writes, "The key is not to prioritize what's on your schedule, but to schedule your priorities." Making time-based goals is all about answering the question "When?"

Putting it all together, an example of a SMART goal might be: *I will exercise at the gym for 30 minutes every Monday, Tuesday, and Thursday. I will go at 5:30 p.m. on the way home from work before I stop at home. To make this possible, I will keep a gym bag in my car with my workout clothes, sneakers, towel, water, and a pre-workout snack.*

Step #4 – Implement

Sam came up with the following SMART behavioral goal(s):

1. Pack his gym bag on Sunday night and keep it by the door so that he'll remember to take it to work with him.

2. On the way home from work on Monday, he will go straight to the gym and work out for 30 minutes.

Once you commit to the SMART goal, the next step is to implement it. When implementing a new strategy, it's important to give the strategy a chance before you fully decide if it works or not. Try not to give up too quickly.

Step #5 – Analyze

As you implement the new SMART goal, think about the experience. What happened? Was there a change? If yes, was it positive or negative? Should you keep this SMART goal or change something?

Sam noticed that he wasn't seeing results. He still found himself wanting to go home after work instead of getting to the gym. So we repeated the process.

Step # 6 – Repeat

Keep following this process until you find strategies that help you reach your goal. That's what Sam did:

(Step #1 – Observe & Reflect)

Me: How were you feeling when you decided to go straight home instead of the gym?

Sam: I was hungry. I hadn't eaten anything since lunch. I didn't want to pass out, and I didn't want to spend money buying something on the way when I already have food at home.

(Step #2 – Brainstorm & Step #3 – Decide)
Me: What do you think will help you get to the gym without having to go home?
Sam: I could pack a snack in my gym bag to eat before I work out.
Me: Awesome! What snack specifically?
Sam: I could pack a banana and an RX bar.

After implementing the strategy and analyzing the results, he was able to get to the gym consistently over the course of the next few months. As simple as it sounds, putting a snack in his gym bag was his key to success.

See if asking yourself these questions can help you identify strategies that might work for your specific situation. If not, you need to dig a little deeper. The answer is always there; it just may be hiding. If you aren't getting the answers you're looking for, then you need to ask yourself better questions.

This is the blueprint for cracking your weight-loss code! While it can seem a bit cumbersome, once you start doing it, it becomes nearly automatic. Will it feel as exciting as buying a cool new system that guarantees you will lose weight quickly and easily? Probably not. But it will feel super exciting at the end, when you start seeing the results it gets you.

Looking For Bright Spots

When trying to achieve a goal, it's common to spend a lot of time focusing on what's going wrong and figuring out how to fix it. While this makes sense on the surface, it can create paralysis by analysis and hinder your confidence.

Instead of just focusing on what's going wrong when observing and reflecting, consider focusing on what's going well. Behavior-change experts call this looking for "bright spots." For example, rather than putting your focus on the food you "shouldn't have eaten," think about a time when you stuck to your eating plan. What could you take from that experience that will help you with this one? What motivated you? What enabled you to make good choices? How were you feeling? Did you make any changes to your schedule? Did you change anything about your environment?

Focusing on these will train your brain to pay closer attention to the positives and guide you to understand what helps you be successful. It will also provide you with great clues, and it might give you the one key piece of the puzzle that you've been looking for.

Tracking Success

I love the saying, "If you don't track it, you won't change it." Cracking your code is about the small details and finding things that do and don't work. When working a case, police detectives keep a notebook on them at all times to jot down thoughts or any vital information that may present itself. You may find it helpful to do the same—especially if you're forgetful like me.

As you do this, look for patterns. For example, many people keep a food journal detailing what they ate, how much they ate, and when they ate it. While this is great, it tells only a small part of the story. You also need to understand triggers, key decisions made during the day, change windows, etc. Remember, if you don't track it, you can't change it, so consider creating a daily discovery journal. If you visit chrisbarlics.com/create-your-own-detectives-journal I lay out the steps to create your own.

The Fickle Scale

What happens when, despite your hard work, the scale doesn't budge? As frustrating as it can be, keep in mind that what you see on the scale, in the moment, may not be indicative of your progress.

First, it is impossible to gain or lose pounds of fat or lean tissue overnight. When you see fast changes on the scale, it has more to do with water weight than anything else. To avoid feeling undue frustration when weighing yourself, here are a few tips.

Number one, weigh yourself at the same time each day. Most choose the morning, before breakfast. That's when your body is in its most dehydrated state, unaffected by recent meals.

Even in the mornings, however, our body weight can fluctuate from day to day for two common reasons: First, we may have had an influx of sodium the night before, causing us to retain water. Second, perhaps we ate so much last night that our body hasn't had the chance to process and digest all of it. In time, both issues will resolve themselves, and your actual weight will show.

Sometimes, though, the scale can start climbing because of dietary changes that have nothing to do with your energy balance. For example, when you're on a low-carb diet, your body stores less glycogen and holds less water in your muscles. Thus, you'll lose a fair amount of weight quickly. But once you start adding carbs back in, your body will hold more water, which could account for as much as a 10-pound swing. While the low-carb strategy can be great for short-term results (if your body can tolerate it), most people start feeling sluggish and depressed and become impulsive. This is why it's so difficult to sustain.

Aside from water weight, other factors can cause the number on the scale to be higher than expected. These include changes in medication, weighing yourself before you go to the bathroom, how much time has passed since you last ate, and the type of food you ate that day.

Because your weight will naturally fluctuate from day to day, instead of focusing on your daily weight, consider focusing on averaging your weight for the week. This will not only enable you to care less about the daily inconsistencies, it will also reflect progress and trends much more accurately.

Non-Scale Methods

The scale is the easiest way to measure progress, but as we've just seen, it can be a bit persnickety. It may be helpful to consider additional ways of measuring success. Since we all define progress differently, how we measure progress should also be an individual thing. Here are a few methods for you to consider:

Take Pictures: Almost all of us have cameras on our phone, making it easy to take progress pictures. Some find it helpful to take these monthly; others like to take them weekly. Your call. Either way, they'll give you a great tool for tracking your progress.

Circumference Measurements: If you don't already have one, buy a simple body tape measure for a few bucks online or at a craft store. Measure any areas that are important to you. To ensure consistency, make sure you measure yourself at the same time each morning, before they can be affected by the day.

Body Fat Percentage: Since it is possible to lose body fat but weigh the same, especially if you're gaining lean muscle, measuring your body-fat percentage can be informative. Unless you're proficient with calipers, measuring this yourself can be tricky. Try finding gyms in your area that can assess your body-fat percentage for you.

Skinny Jeans: How your clothes feel—whether it's a favorite dress, suit, or your skinny jeans—can also be great signs of progress.

Cracking Your Code One Piece At A Time

Cracking your code doesn't happen all at once. A lot of patience and good detective work is required. Success is the result of repeatedly identifying the next skill and behavior to improve and finding a way to improve it. It's about brainstorming ideas, choosing which one(s) to implement, tracking your results and adjusting according to the findings.

It can be helpful to think of the process like putting together a puzzle - it happens piece by piece. Once you have a vision for what your puzzle should look like, you start by finding the first two pieces that fit together and build out from there. Along the way, you'll find some pieces will be obvious and fit on the first try. Other times you may have to try several pieces until you find the one that fits. Often, cracking the code is about finding one or two tiny but pivotal pieces that bring the whole puzzle together. The key to cracking your code is to not get discouraged - to keep trying different pieces until you find the ones that fit together. Remember, if it was easy, everyone would do it.

Key Points

- Finding the tools, strategies and resources you need to be successful is a task that only you can complete.

- The process of cracking your code is about trial and learning - requiring a lot of patience.

- To find what works for you, consider using the iteration cycle.

- Asking yourself quality questions will result in quality answers. Keep digging deeper!

- By focusing first on discovering key change and decision windows during your day/week, you will be more likely to identify pivotal strategies that will help you reach your goal.

- When creating a strategy, make sure it is Specific, Measurable, Actionable, Realistic, and Time-based.

- When searching for answers, rather than focusing on what's going wrong, think about times when things went right - even briefly. What lessons can you learn from those experiences and apply going forward?

- Sometimes it can hard to remember the "a-ha" moments. Keeping a journal will allow you to keep track of important discoveries, thoughts, and future strategies to try.

- It's hard to change what you cannot measure. Find a way to track your progress that works for you - it doesn't just have to be the scale.

PART 3: THE OPTIONS

Skills, Concepts And Strategies To Consider When Brainstorming

Chapter 6

Considerations For Controlling Caloric Intake

"When you improve a little each day, eventually big things occur. Don't look for the big, quick improvement. Seek the small improvement one day at a time. That's the only way it happens – and when it happens, it lasts." -*John Wooden*

The two biggest factors for achieving nutritional success are creating a plan that gives you results (i.e., feeling and looking good) and that is sustainable. This chapter will give you many ideas that will help you do just that.

Part of sustainability is not feeling restricted. For example, let's say 1,700 Calories was your target Caloric intake for a particular day, but just a cheeseburger, large fries, and a milkshake would put you above your target. That's only one meal! So how do you get your best bang for your Calorie buck?

A vital key to staying within your Calorie allotment without feeling restricted (or lightheaded and lacking energy) is to consume more nutrient-dense food than Calorie-dense food. Nutrient-dense foods are packed with nutrients without a ton of Calories. Not only will eating these allow you to eat more food to reach your Calories, they'll keep you fuller longer—especially if you also choose foods that are high in protein and/or fiber—so that your cravings won't be crazy.

Nutrient-dense foods include salmon, chicken breast, cod, mussels, oysters, cucumbers, oatmeal, grapefruit, strawberries, peaches, honeydew melon, lettuce, popcorn, beans, lentils, mozzarella cheese, Greek yogurt, and almond milk—to name just a few.

However, if you ignore this option and eat mostly Calorie-dense foods, you will find you deplete your Calorie allotment a lot quicker. How will you know the difference? Well, cheeseburgers, French fries, donuts, pizza, desserts, and baked goods are all considered Calorie-dense foods (foods high in Calories for the amount of food you're eating).

While these may seem obvious, certain seemingly healthy foods can also be very Calorie-dense. These include fruit juices, nuts, avocados, dried fruits, dairy products, fatty cuts of meat, and Starbucks coffee. Remember, you can be eating healthy and still gain weight! At the end of the day, it's all about Calories in compared to Calories out.

Am I suggesting you cut out Calorie-dense foods completely? Of course not! Being successful is not about restriction. It's about recognizing how many Calories these foods contain and, if these foods are important to you, figuring out ways to work them into a plan that makes sense for you.

Liquid Calories

Success requires being mindful not only of what we eat, but also what we drink. It can be easy to overlook liquid Calories. Having a glass of orange juice for breakfast, an iced tea for lunch, and soda for dinner can add up to 350 Calories—assuming you had only one eight-ounce glass of each. Since the average glass size is 10–12 ounces, that's a big assumption. Twelve ounces of each per day would bump it up over 500 Calories.

Certain drinks can be 500 Calories by themselves. A Venti-iced Frappuccinos at Starbucks averages a little over 500 Calories each. Even the seemingly healthy Venti Green Tea Frappuccino has the same number of Calories as two slices of pizza! But that's not the worst. The popular large (32-ounce) Dunkin' Donuts Frozen Mocha Coffee Coolatta is 990 Calories! A small version comes in around 300 Calories.

Again I'm not suggesting you cut these out completely. I'm suggesting you act like a detective and research the Calorie content so that you can be more mindful about what you put in your mouth.

Diet Soda

On the surface, diet soda seems like a good idea. You can enjoy drinking a soda without any of the Calories. However, there does seem to be a correlation between diet soda and weight gain. While much more research still needs to be done, preliminary thought is that artificial sweeteners in diet drinks can actually increase our cravings by throwing off our body's ability to regulate satiety, thus causing us to eat more. Basically, when our brain senses something sweet, it expects Calories to come with it. When they don't, our metabolism gets thrown for a loop.

Like anything else, if you drink diet soda, don't shoot the messenger! Put your detective's hat on to see if you notice patterns that point to diet soda increasing your cravings or decreasing your energy. If you do, act accordingly.

Alcohol

Alcohol is a big contributing factor to weight gain for many people as it has seven Calories per gram. Four ounces of red wine is 95 kcal, and a 12-ounce glass of beer averages between 125 and 150 Calories. One glass is all well and good, but when drinking alcohol, one glass can turn into three or four pretty quickly.

Mixed drinks are another story. One regular eight-ounce margarita averages 455 Calories, while a 12-ounce margarita can contain as many as 680 Calories. A night out consuming two to three of these can really derail your weight-loss efforts.

When it comes to our health-and-fitness journey, consider also that the adverse effects of alcohol go beyond just its Calorie count. Alcohol lowers inhibition, making us more likely to indulge in Calorie-dense foods that we find at parties and bars. And when we eat while drinking alcohol, the fat-burning process is hindered because our bodies use the Calories from alcohol first as fuel.

Water

If you're like many Americans, water is not your drink of choice. But according to research, in addition to saving you hundreds of Calories per day, drinking eight to 10 eight-ounce glasses of water daily can boost your metabolism as well as decrease your appetite. If you are considering adding more water to your diet, here are a few ways that can help:

Sometimes going back and forth to fill an eight-ounce glass can be tedious and time-consuming. Instead, try using a 16–24-ounce water bottle. It is sometimes less overwhelming to think about drinking three bottles of water than eight to 10 glasses.

Drink a glass of water before every meal. Not only will it help you drink more water, studies also show drinking a glass of water before eating decreases your appetite.

Sometimes the hunger you're feeling is really thirst, so before you reach for that snack, drink a glass of water. If your hunger goes away, you know you were only thirsty, and you saved a few hundred Calories.

Drink cold water. According to a study published in the Journal of Endocrinology & Metabolism, researchers found drinking cold water can boost your metabolic rate by 30 percent. That's an extra 100 Calories if you drink eight to 10 glasses of cold water per day!

Watch Out For Sneaky Calories

If we're going to track our Calorie intake, we need to be careful that we're accounting for ALL Calories. Some aren't as obvious as others, and these "sneaky" Calories can unknowingly add 300–500 extra Calories per day. Here are some examples:

When counting the toast, don't forget to count the butter or jelly.

When counting the coffee, don't forget the sugar or creamer.

When counting the salad, don't forget to count the dressing.

When counting the Greek yogurt, don't forget to count the granola/ fruit.

When counting the chicken or salmon, don't forget to count the sauce.

When counting the sandwich, don't forget to count the condiments.

When counting the chips, don't forget to count the dip/salsa.

When counting the fries, don't forget to count the ketchup.

When counting the pasta, don't forget to count the sauce (or the gravy if you're Italian).

When counting the entrée, don't forget to count the sides.

When counting the pancakes, don't forget to count the butter/syrup.

When counting the cereal, don't forget to count the milk.

When counting the food, don't forget to count the beverages.

Also, when cooking, don't forget to account for the spoonfuls of food you "taste." These can also quickly add up.

A "Little Of This" Can Add Up To A Lot

According to research, approximately 25 percent of our total Calories come from snacking. This means if you consistently go over your target, there's a possibility that the extra Calories come from snacking. First, let me say again, there's nothing wrong with snacking. It's only an issue if overdoing it causes you to go over your daily Calorie goals and it's something you'd like to change.

If it is, the first step is to identify your change and decision windows (see the previous chapter). For many, snacking is especially common during the second half of the day. This includes at work after lunch, when you get home from work, before dinner, and, of course, nighttime snacking after dinner.

Once you've identified your window, next investigate some possible options. If, for example, excessive snacking between lunch and dinner is an issue, consider what you're eating for breakfast and especially lunch. Are you getting adequate protein and fiber in these meals? Are you eating breakfast at all?

I don't believe in universal dietary rules because everyone is different. There are many people who do well without eating breakfast. For them, forcing something down in the morning would just add meaningless Calories to their day. However, if you feel ravenous in the afternoon, you might want to test what happens if you do eat different types of foods for breakfast. Does it make you less hungry throughout the day?

I don't want to imply that an afternoon snack is bad and should be avoided. For many of us, it would be asking a lot to go from 12:30 p.m. to dinner without eating something. A wholesome snack in the afternoon is great, as long as you plan these extra Calories into your day.

Read the last half of that last sentence again. You need to plan ahead. What snack would you like to plan into your afternoon? Where will you get it? Will you bring it from home? I ask because unless you're lucky, the vending-machine snacks at work tend to be Calorie-dense and will leave you starving a few hours later.

Another common change window for a lot of people, including many of my clients, is when they come home from work, when they would snack on "a little of this" or "a little of that" before dinner. Remember, a few handfuls of pretzels and/or nuts plus a granola bar can quickly add up to several hundred extra Calories each day.

If this is you, remember that you will only snack on the foods you keep in the house. If you want to stop snacking between the time when you get home and when you eat dinner, perhaps the answer is not keeping Calorie-dense snacks in the house. Or, perhaps, eating more protein or fiber earlier in the day will alleviate your desire to snack when you get home. Or maybe the key lies in eating a more nutrient-dense snack.

Eating Out

I'm Italian, which means eating out is one of my favorite pastimes. I love spending time with friends and family, enjoying the ambiance and, obviously, the delicious food. But if we're not careful, dining out can derail our weight-loss efforts by creating a huge Calorie surplus.

It is staggering how many Calories we can unknowingly consume when dining out. One meal could contain your whole daily Calorie allotment! Here's a quick example:

Let's say you go out for dinner and you start with a glass of wine or soda—that's 125–150 Calories per glass. For the sake of keeping the count on the low side, let's say you have only one glass per meal. Next, you have only one dinner roll from the bread basket. That's around 270 Calories; add butter and it becomes 320 Calories (butter is 100 Calories per tablespoon). Then comes the appetizer, which usually contains 600–800 Calories on average. Next is the side salad, which is at least 100 Calories, but it can be more, depending on the dressing.

We're at 1,270 Calories, and we haven't even gotten to the entree yet! Speaking of, the average entree is around 900 Calories. Then comes many people's undoing, the dessert. If you top off your great meal with a piece of chocolate cake, that's at least another 350 Calories.

The grand total for this meal is over 2,500 Calories! That's assuming you had only one glass of wine/soda, ate only one roll, and didn't order the more Calorie-dense appetizers, entrees, or desserts. Even if you were conservative and consumed only 800 Calories earlier in the day, your Calorie count for that day would still be 3,300!

Doing this twice per week, even if you stick to a 1,500-Calorie diet the remaining five days of the week, would still bring your average daily intake for the week to 2,015 kcal. If your Caloric expenditure number was a little over 2,000, these two nights of overeating per week could be the difference between losing one pound a week and losing nothing at all.

If you're like me and you love dining out but don't want to kill your results, here are a few strategies you can try:

- Researchers found that those who drank alcohol before a meal ate almost 200 Calories more than those who didn't. This is because alcohol boosts short-term appetite and temporarily blocks our body's ability to feel full. It can also lower our inhibitions. For most people, however, this can take a little while to go into effect. So if you want to have that glass of wine at the restaurant but want to minimize the damage, consider waiting until after the bread and appetizers are off the table to order your Pinot.

- Research found that those who ate bread before their meal consumed an average of 16 percent more Calories. When we eat one piece of bread, it's usually followed by a second and then a fourth. If you wish to avoid this, try moving the bread so that it isn't within arm's reach. You can either send it away or move it to the other end of the table.

- Look at the menu and plan your meal ahead of time so that you're not tempted by the menu in the moment.

- If possible, stick with water or just one glass of wine.

- Enter the restaurant well hydrated (thirst sometimes feels like hunger).

- Order your entree from the appetizer menu.

- Avoid dessert altogether; they tend to be the most Calorie-dense.

- Eat slowly.

- Ask for a "doggy bag" as soon as your meal comes and immediately put half the portion into it for the next day.

The one tip I absolutely want you to consider is that, when you do go out, enjoy yourself! Utilizing the strategies above will help you avoid sabotaging your results, but don't let them keep you from having a good time or enjoying your food.

Beware of the Halo

Have you ever heard of "halo"? No, not Halo Ice Cream (which is a great low-Calorie ice cream option, by the way). I'm talking about something called the "halo effect." It's when seeing certain key phrases such as "healthy," "organic," "fat-free," or "gluten-free" justifies our desire to indulge. It typically sounds like this, "These cookies are gluten-free so I can have more because they're healthy."

My wife, Patrice, has a gluten allergy and often buys gluten-free cookies called K-Toos. They're basically the gluten-free equivalent of Oreos and are equally as addicting. Several times I have caught myself thinking, "They're gluten-free. I can have two or three more." The implication is that because they are gluten-free, they must be okay.

Research shows that foods labeled "healthy" often are higher in Calories than others. Those K-too cookies are 60 Calories per cookie, compared to only 45 in Oreos. This is nothing new. In 1992 there was something researchers called the "SnackWell syndrome," where people consumed large amounts of SnackWell's cookies because they were labeled fat-free.

Do you have any "magic words" that make you more likely to indulge? Being mindful and aware of this is the best weapon to help you take control and avoid this from happening.

Slow Down

Nowadays, we try to cram as much into our days as possible. Our schedules are crazy, and we try to do everything quickly, including eating. Gobbling down our food, however, can have major consequences on both our health and our waistline.

Studies have shown that those who eat slower often eat less. Eating slower can help us cut down our intake for several reasons. First, it takes about twenty minutes for satiety hormones (leptin and neuropeptide Y) to reach our brain, letting us know we're full. If we eat fast, we'll consume more food during those twenty minutes.

Eating slowly also enables your body to better digest and metabolize food. Digestion starts in the mouth with enzymes contained in our saliva. The slower we eat, the more time we have to chew. The more we chew our food, the less our stomach has to work, which leads to better nutrient absorption and metabolism and fewer digestive issues. In a perfect world, we'd chew each bite between ten and twenty times.

Perhaps the best benefit of eating slower is that it enables us to actually savor and enjoy what we are eating. Many of us don't just eat—we eat and talk, eat and watch TV, eat and do work. We even eat and drive. This mindless eating not only makes us consume far more Calories, it also diminishes the enjoyment we get from eating.

How fast do you eat? If you think it may be too fast, here are some strategies to help you slow down. The first one is to put your fork down between bites. After taking a bite, breathe. Focus on the smell of the food, enjoy the texture, and savor the taste. Experience and enjoy the food you're eating rather than immediately thinking about the next bite.

If you pay attention, you'll find that after the first few bites, the enjoyment of eating usually starts to diminish. Instead of focusing on eating fast and finishing whatever is in front of us, slow down and stop eating when you stop enjoying the food. Is the second half of that cookie worth the extra Calories? Is finishing your entire plate of pasta worth it?

Here are a few more strategies that may help you put the brakes on speed eating:

- Sip water in between bites.

- Use chopsticks.

- Sit down to eat instead of standing. When you stand, you are usually eating quicker to move on to doing something else.

- Don't wait until you're super hungry to eat. When you're ravenous, you'll be more likely to eat quickly.

- Another strategy is to change hands. According to research, using your non-dominant hand when eating snack food can cut your consumption by up to 30 percent. The reason? Eating with your non-dominant hand prevents mindless eating.

Consistency

Ultimately, the best diet for us is going to be the one we stick to. We shouldn't have to choose between sustainability and effectiveness. The key is to create a nutritional strategy that works that is also sustainable. But it's not black or white.

Our progress is dictated by what we do 90 percent of the time, not what we do on special occasions. Let's say you eat 35 times during the week (three meals and two snacks multiplied by seven days/week). Your success is not determined by two or three of those meals; it's determined by what you do during the other 32 or 33. It is determined by your daily breakfasts, lunches, and dinners. The afternoon and late-night snacks. The type of beverages you consume. These are what really matter.

When you go out with friends or family, that is not the time to worry about your progress. It's a time to enjoy having fun with the people that make your life worth living.

I've spoken to too many people who will go out to dinner and put all their focus on not having the bread, not having an appetizer while everyone else does, not having dessert, and ordering just a grilled shrimp salad. When it's over, they realize that they didn't even enjoy themselves and they go home and binge on cookies, ice cream, and chips because they spent so much mental energy "being good" at the restaurant. It would have been better if they ate a piece of bread and shared an appetizer or a dessert—especially if they only go out to dinner once per week.

Now, I'm not saying to go out and consume 2,500 Calories in one sitting on these special occasions (unless we're talking about Thanksgiving), but I am saying that it's okay to not always be in Calorie-counting mode. Have an idea of what you're eating (the more you get in the habit of counting Calories and gaining awareness, the more you can make accurate guesstimates about what you're eating), don't be super strict, listen to your body, and get back on track immediately after. While it isn't always easy, losing weight should not be a miserable process. If it is, you're doing it wrong!

The Root Of The Problem

Sometimes, what seems like the problem can really just be a symptom of a deeper problem. This is often the case with food. I don't feel like I would be doing you justice if, on your journey, I didn't end this section by asking you to consider whether you have deeper reasons for overeating than what we've discussed so far. A popular acronym that may help is the HALT method:

Hunger – It is normal to feel hungry when your body needs to eat. However, if you find that you're constantly hungry, this could mean you're body is hungry for nourishment. Perhaps you're deficient in essential vitamins or minerals. Perhaps you're not eating enough nutrient-dense foods. If you think this may be the case, seeking guidance from a doctor or registered dietician would be recommended. But sometimes, what appears to be hunger may actually be something else.

Anxiety – Many people use food as a stress-reliever - a way to calm themselves or make up for things that they're not happy about (regarding themselves, their lives or a difficult life situation). For some, food is the only thing they feel they can look forward to during their day. If, after doing some investigating, you realize you are using food as a coping mechanism, then working on the underlying issues becomes key. In Chapter 10, I provide some proven strategies for relieving stress, but if you find they aren't enough, consider seeking guidance from a mental health practitioner. This does not make you "broken" or weak. On the contrary, it makes you a good detective willing to do what's necessary to crack your code (be healthy and happy).

Loneliness– Feeling isolated and bored are two of the most common reasons people overeat. If you feel one of these applies to you, perhaps reaching out to someone will help. Make a phone call, visit a coworker's cubicle, or reach out to someone via social media. See if this decreases your urge to eat. I recognize this is much easier said than done, so spend some time brainstorming and experimenting with possible strategies that you feel can help.

Tired/Thirst – As we've already discussed, thirst can mimic hunger. Try drinking a glass of water and see if your hunger subsides.

However, if you are tired, this may also increase your hunger hormones. Getting the proper amount of sleep can help keep your appetite in check (more on this in Chapter 10).

Key Points

- Eating more Nutrient-dense foods will allow you to eat more food without going over your Calorie goals.

- Not all Calories are from food. Make sure you factor in liquid Calories.

- For accuracy when counting Calories, make sure you include snacking, toppings, and "little bites and tastes" when you're cooking.

- If you enjoy eating out, plan ahead so you can enjoy yourself without sabotaging your results.

- Try slowing down and savoring the food that you're eating. Eating too fast will cause you to consume more Calories and limit your enjoyment of the meal.

- The key to success is consistency - it's not about what you do occasionally that matters, it's what you do day in and day out that counts.

- Cracking your code to create long-term nutritional success depends on you finding and treating the underlying cause(s) of overeating - sometimes it's much more complicated than just simple hunger or awareness of portion control.

Chapter 7

Strategies For Increasing Caloric Expenditure

"We do not stop exercising because we grow old - we grow old because we stop exercising." -Kenneth Cooper

On October 16, 2010, the Rutgers University football team played the Army football team at MetLife Stadium. With five minutes left in the fourth quarter, junior defensive tackle Eric LeGrand ran down the field during a kickoff in hopes of making a play. At 270 pounds of muscle, he ran as fast as his powerful legs could take him, and as the receiver made the catch, he left his feet to make the tackle. He had no way of knowing that his life was about to change forever. Upon impact, he went headfirst into the receiver, fracturing his C3 and C4 vertebrae, immediately paralyzing him from the neck down.

Nine years later, turning tragedy into triumph, Eric LeGrand has become an author, motivational speaker, and poster child for never giving up. However, despite all he's accomplished, he continues to dedicate his life to one particular goal—regaining the ability to walk on his own. Initially, doctors gave him a 0–5 percent chance that this would ever happen. Despite seemingly insurmountable odds, Eric continues to work diligently to make his goal a reality and is slowly making progress.

Eric LeGrand is an inspiration—not only to never give up, but to appreciate the small things, like our ability to move our body freely and independently. How often do we take this ability for granted—to stand up and walk where we want to, when we want to, as fast or slow as we want to? Think about what life would be like if you lost this ability.

I bet that if Eric were given the ability to walk, he wouldn't sit for 12 or more hours a day, the way so many of us do. That's because he has a unique perspective. Here is a brave young man, who, at the prime of his life, had his body taken away from him. Now, his biggest dream is not to win the lottery or to be a movie star … it's to move his arms and legs.

More than those of us who can move our arms and legs, he appreciates the fundamental purpose of exercise. It's not about burning Calories. Exercise is about celebrating what your body can do and making it stronger so that you can live able-bodied and independently well into your eighties, nineties, and beyond. It's about being able to go explore a new place, play with children and grandchildren, and go for a long walk on the beach. If you're moving, you're alive, and the more you move, the more alive you'll feel.

Many of us who are able-bodied are wasting the gift we've been given. We live a sedentary lifestyle, effectively living much of our day as if we too were paralyzed. Life gets hectic. We become so focused on earning a living, raising a family, and trying to keep up with all life throws at us that exercise can fall low on our priority list. But if we're not careful, we too may lose our ability to move freely and independently, leaving us regretting we didn't take better care of ourselves when we had the chance.

The Problem

Many people watch their bodies break down slowly over time, some due to age, but more often from a lack of proper physical activity. Half a century ago, our way of life was different, and it was much easier to be physically active. Today, so much in our world revolves around sitting. Desk jobs, smartphones, Amazon, Uber, and on-demand entertainment make the need for physical activity almost obsolete. We view going for a walk, running outside, and moving around as superfluous chores, rather than a privilege.

For years, we have been bombarded with a constant barrage of messaging comprised of two central themes. The first has to do with why we need to exercise. The second can best be summed up by the phrase "no pain, no gain." In other words, you need to punish yourself physically to see results.

Clearly these strategies haven't worked as 80–90 percent of us are not getting the minimum recommended amount of physical activity. Fear might compel us to get started, but for most, it is not a sustainable source of motivation. And if you view exercise as a form of punishment for what you've eaten, you're always going to find reasons to escape it.

Focus On What You'll Gain (Not Lose) From Exercising

If one of your goals is to add more exercise to your life, it's important to first ask yourself, "Why?" Many people would say that it will help them burn more Calories, resulting in weight loss.

Will consistent physical activity burn Calories and help you lose weight? Yes, but exercise alone will not help you create sustainable weight loss. When people set out to exercise thinking that it alone will help them lose weight, they are setting false expectations that inevitably lead to frustration and giving up. After exercising for a period of time, if the scale doesn't move as much as they hoped, they stop exercising. This is because exercise doesn't burn as many Calories as most people think.

Here is a list of common forms of physical activity and how many Calories (approximately) someone weighing 185 pounds would burn doing 30 minutes of that activity:

Weight Lifting (general): 133 Calories

Water Aerobics: 178 Calories

Tai Chi: 178 Calories

Walking (3.5 mph): 178 Calories

Stationary Bike (moderate): 211 Calories

Dancing: 244 Calories

Low-Impact Aerobics: 244 Calories

Weight Lifting (vigorous): 266 Calories

Swimming (general): 266 Calories

High-Impact Aerobics: 311 Calories

Rowing (moderate): 311 Calories

Circuit Training: 355 Calories

Running (12 min/mile): 355 Calories

Elliptical (moderate): 400 Calories

Stair-Step Machine (general): 400 Calories

Martial Arts: 444 Calories

When figuring out how to crack your code, remember that you can't out exercise a poor diet; you would have to work yourself to the bone in order to come close. Even if you did, your body would never be able to sustain that pace for long, and it would hurt your metabolism and health in the process (more on this a little later). This is a bit of a generalization, but ask yourself what seems more doable—substituting a Starbucks Frappuccino for a regular cup of coffee in the morning or running four miles each day? Both would save you almost 500 Calories, but which one is more realistic for you?

If you're thinking, "Then what's the point of exercising if it doesn't burn that many Calories?" then stay with me and consider this: when it comes to adding exercise as a consistent part of your life, what if you focused on what you'll gain from it rather than what you could lose? Exercise has a tremendous number of benefits. Yes, exercise can support long-term weight loss if it's done correctly (see the "Increasing Your Metabolism" section later in this chapter). It also greatly reduces our risk of cancer, diabetes, heart disease, and falling. It improves our sleep quality, energy, mood, and flexibility; AND it gives us better bone health, increased longevity, improved cognition, increased productivity, greater endurance, and more strength—just to name a few.

In other words, physical activity helps us live a longer, more enjoyable life! Unfortunately, many don't understand this until it's too late— until being sedentary creates irreparable damage and we're looking back regretting that we didn't start sooner. Remember, the key is to connect with the reasons you want to exercise, not why you think you should.

What's The Best Exercise Program?

When it comes to exercise, everybody wants to know the best, most effective type that will provide the biggest bang for their effort. There are equally as many exercise programs out there as diet plans—everything from CrossFit, Pilates, and barre classes, to yoga, high-intensity interval training (HIIT), and regular old steady-state training.

Similar to eating strategies, it's important to accept that there is no one best way to exercise. Everything works, but not everything will work for you. Some may not be the right intensity, others may bore you, and certain programs may not help you with what you want to achieve. Ultimately, the best exercise program for you is the one you will stick with consistently. To find out which one that is, consider the "3E model." For an exercise program to work for you, it probably needs to be some combination of effective, efficient, and enjoyable.

Effective

How do you know if the exercise you're doing is effective? Some say a workout is only effective if it makes you sore. While we've all heard the no-pain, no-gain approach before, numerous amounts of data have shown that muscle soreness is not a reliable indicator of a good workout.

To understand why, it first helps to understand what soreness is. The most common form is known as delayed-onset muscle soreness (DOMS), which is caused by micro trauma in the muscles and surrounding tissue, resulting in inflammation and stiffness lasting 24–72 hours. Although it is normal to experience this after you do a new exercise or something you haven't done in a while, your body should soon adapt, and you will gradually become less sore following a workout.

When the soreness subsides, does that mean the workout is no longer effective? No! It simply means your body is better conditioned for exercise. It doesn't mean you need to change things up to create muscle confusion because confused muscles often get injured. Should you never change your workout? Of course not! After a month or two, you can progress your stage of training or type of program, but it's always advisable to consult with a trainer for the best way to do this.

Okay, so if soreness isn't a good indicator, how can you tell if your workouts are effective? The answer is one word: progress. Are you seeing results? Unfortunately, a lot of people stop exercising because they think they're not making any progress. If your only measure of progress is the scale, you're bound to get frustrated.

Perhaps, instead of focusing on the scale, consider focusing first on the small improvements you make along the way. After a few workouts, are you able to do a few more reps? Are you able to lift a little more weight? Are you feeling a little less tired when you walk or run? Are your muscles feeling a little looser? These are all indicators that you're on the right path. Small achievements quickly add up to long-term goal attainment.

It's not just about how much weight you lose. How do you feel? How do your clothes fit? What effect is exercise having on your stamina, on your strength, and on your mobility? Don't worry about speed or intensity. At first, consistency is the name of the game. Regardless of how slow you go, you're still lapping those who stay on the couch. However, if you're not seeing progress after working out for a few weeks, if you're feeling weaker, stiffer, and more fatigued, then something is wrong. You should seek additional guidance.

Remember, exercise is about building yourself up and feeling good, not kicking the crap out of yourself to the point of exhaustion. Doing that only leads to mental and physical burnout and the release of a cascade of stress hormones (which contribute to fat storage, not burning); it can also lead to injury.

Efficiency

Efficiency, by definition, is about achieving maximum productivity with little wasted effort. Something can be enjoyable and effective, but if it takes a lot of preparation (an hour drive to the hiking trail), you're unlikely to do it consistently. Efficiency is about many things. First, it's about eliminating the steps you need to take to get started. It shouldn't take 30 minutes to get ready to exercise. If it does, you'll be more likely to opt out.

It should also be doable. In other words, it should not require resources you do not or cannot have at your disposal. If, for example, you enjoy boxing and feel it would be effective for you but you do not have a place to box, this would obviously be your first problem to solve.

If You Don't Enjoy What You're Doing, You're Doing The Wrong Thing

The final E is arguably the most important if you want to be consistent with exercise. We've been conditioned to think of exercise as more of a punishment than something enjoyable, as if it is the debt we need to pay for all the bad food we have eaten. People will often tell you how much, how often, how hard, or what type of exercise you "should do," and if you don't like it, you just need to "suck it up." If you keep following this belief system, you're going to fail.

The prevailing belief about exercise is that if you're not drenched in sweat and pushing yourself hard for an hour each and every single day, then you won't reach your goal. This is just not true. We humans instinctually run away from things that make us uncomfortable and seek out comfort. So if the no-pain, no-gain approach to exercise doesn't sound fun to you, then perhaps you need to listen to yourself. It doesn't make you a wuss; it makes you self-aware and intelligent.

Consider starting by finding a form of exercise you enjoy. A great way to begin is to think back and ask yourself if there was ever a form of physical activity you used to like. It could be anything—dancing, kickboxing, yoga, going for walks, etc. If there was something you used to do, see if there's a way for you to add it back into your life. Everything counts!

If you're thinking, "What if I don't like any form of exercise?" then consider finding an activity that sucks the least. For example, if you hate running, don't run! The one-mile walk you do consistently is always better than the one-mile run you never do. Trying to do something you hate is always a failing strategy. Instead, investigate and find something that brings you at least a little joy.

Expenditure Is About More Than Exercise

While exercise is the most controllable method of expending Calories, if you want to understand all the components of weight loss, then there are other factors to consider. As a reminder, increasing your Caloric expenditure is about increasing the following three things:

1. Your metabolism
2. Your thermic effect of feeding
3. Your physical activity

What follows are some ideas to consider for increasing the first two. As always, it's up to you to think about how these may be applicable to you.

Increasing Your Metabolism

In Chapter 4, we discussed that our metabolism accounts for 50–70 percent of our daily Caloric expenditure. In addition to keeping our weight and body fat down, a well-functioning metabolism means our body is getting the energy it needs, is detoxing properly, and is repairing tissues and that our hormones are functioning properly. Basically it means we feel happy and healthy.

Shockingly, what many have been told to do to lose weight actually slows our metabolism. The common philosophy of eating only 1,200 Calories, cutting out certain food groups (like carbs and all sugar), and doing tons of cardio might create initial weight loss, but none of it is sustainable—and it is often metabolically damaging.

The more and more we go on these crash diets, the lower our BMR goes, which is why diets literally make it harder for us to lose weight. These diets damage our mitochondria and decrease cellular respiration. This means that low-Calorie diets and seemingly healthy detoxes often deprive our cells of proper nutrients, damaging them and decreasing our metabolism. Detoxes and cleanses may initially make us feel good, but it's because we aren't eating the processed crap we normally eat—not because of the special shakes we purchase. Remember, our body has a natural mechanism for detoxing—our liver and kidneys!

Mitochondrial damage—and thus metabolic damage—is also caused by overly stressful exercise. An example would be long-duration cardio that leaves us exhausted. While you may burn some Calories, you are also depleting muscle and lowering your BMR. On the contrary, burst or interval training has been shown to be metabolically supportive.

Research has also shown that the more lean muscle you have, the higher your basal metabolic rate. Thus, while appropriate cardiovascular exercise has many health benefits, if increasing your BMR is your goal, consider incorporating more weight training as well. Contrary to what many fear, it will not make you bulky (muscle doesn't grow that fast).

When we create an energy deficit solely by cutting Calories, without any exercise, approximately 25–33 percent of weight loss is from muscle. Burning muscle lowers our metabolism (the more muscle we have, the higher our BMR tends to be). It's the exercise equivalent of "being penny-wise and dollar-foolish." Long-term weight loss success with exercise isn't about how many Calories you burn during a workout; it's mainly about building lean muscle to positively affect your basal metabolic rate.

However, proper exercise is not the only strategy for boosting your metabolism. Additional strategies include getting adequate sleep, increasing your vitamin D (through food, supplementation, or sunlight), and increasing your intake of metabolically supportive foods. What types of foods? Shellfish, organic eggs, grass-fed beef, white fish, organic beef broth, liver, organic dairy, organic fruits (e.g., pineapple, squash, tomatoes, melons, cherries, grapes, apples, pears, and peaches), organic vegetables (e.g., carrots, zucchini, and potatoes), and organic dark chocolate are all good examples.

On flip side, foods that are metabolically damaging include white bread, farmed beef, foods with high fructose corn syrup (e.g., soda), trans fats such as margarine, soy, polyunsaturated fatty acids (e.g., vegetable oils), and most fried or processed foods.

I cannot say it enough: every body is different. The key word in this book is EXPERIMENTATION. You may find it helpful to keep a food journal and see how changes in food affect your mood, energy, cognition, and health.

Increasing Your Thermic Effect Of Feeding

Another part of the bigger picture is understanding your TEF and how to increase it, which is all about creating the right macronutrient ratio. Whole foods and foods with higher amounts of protein have a higher TEF. For example, your body burns 20–30 percent of the total Calories eaten from protein for digestion, while it burns only 5–10 percent of the Calories eaten from carbs and 0–3 percent from foods high in fat.

This means that if you eat 100 Calories from protein, your body uses 20–30 of those Calories to digest and absorb the protein, leaving you with a net of 70–80 Calories. Pure carbohydrate would leave you with a net 90–95 Calories, and fat would give you a net 97–100 Calories. So a diet higher in protein could mean burning as many as 50–60 Calories more per day. While this doesn't make a huge difference, it has the equivalent Caloric expenditure of walking an extra half a mile each day.

It is also worth noting that in addition to triggering us to eat more, processed foods decrease our TEF by as much as 50 percent compared to whole foods. In other words, our body burns more Calories digesting whole foods than it does processed foods. This could mean a swing of 100 Calories or more in the wrong direction. This is just another reason we may want to stay away from processed foods with ingredients we can't pronounce and, instead, consider eating more foods that come straight from nature.

Important Clue: Not only is it helpful to realize that the types of food we eat affect how much energy we expend digesting food, but it has been well established that eating foods higher in protein and fiber also keep us fuller longer. Foods higher in protein and fiber tend to be less Calorie-dense, which means we can eat more actual food and still lose weight.

Key Points

- Physical activity is not about punishing yourself to lose weight. It is about celebrating what our body can do and staying physically independent so you don't become a prisoner in your own body.

- The "no pain, no gain" approach to exercise is factually inaccurate and creates a perception that exercise has to hurt in order to be effective.

- Exercise has a number of benefits aside from weight loss.

- Physical activity should not be used as a long-term strategy to compensate for a poor eating strategies. Nobody can out-exercise a poor diet for very long.

- Finding the best exercise program for you is about finding one that is efficient, effective and is enjoyable.

- Remember, expenditure is about much more than burning Calories through exercise. It is also about our Metabolism (BMR) and our Thermic Effect of Feeding.

- Many traditional weight loss strategies damage our Metabolism and thus, make it harder to lose weight in the long-term. Instead, consider focusing on incorporating strategies that will give your metabolism a boost.

- By eating more natural and whole foods, we will increase our Thermic Effect of Feeding.

Chapter 8

Motivation

"Only I can change my life. No one can do it for me." -Carol Burnett

Have you ever lost the motivation to do something? I'm going to go out on a limb and assume you have. Virtually everyone who has tried losing weight is familiar with the frustrating cycle of on-again, off-again motivation. Sometimes we can find motivation easily, while at other times, it can feel like we don't care. It can make you feel lazy or even broken, but let me assure you that feeling like you aren't motivated is quite normal.

There are a lot of "rah-rah" answers for increasing motivation. People tell us, "You just need to make it a priority" or, "You just need to try harder." There are no quick fixes for motivation, but we can certainly strengthen it. Before we discuss helpful strategies for increasing motivation, let's first gain some insight about what motivation actually is.

What Is Motivation Exactly?

Motivation is the mental energy that drives us to want to do something and causes us to take action. This should not be confused with willpower, which is the mental energy we use to act (or not act) in opposition to our immediate desires (e.g., not eating that delicious cake in front of us OR wanting to binge-watch our favorite shows but instead choosing to get off the couch to exercise). We'll discuss willpower in the next chapter, but for now, it's important to note the distinction between it and motivation.

When we say we're motivated to do something, at that moment we're not making a huge effort to do it, but we have crossed some sort of mental threshold and now WANT to do the behavior in question. For example, if you're really motivated to exercise, at that moment you really desire to exercise.

Enjoyment isn't the only source for motivation, however; it can also spring from a feeling of necessity. As the saying goes, "Change happens when the pain of staying the same is greater than the pain of change." Motivation works in much the same way. Perhaps we have been putting off adding more exercise into our lives or making a change to our diet. Eventually, we weigh the cost of taking action vs. the cost of doing nothing and realize that doing nothing seems like the more painful option. Thus, we become motivated to act.

Weighing Your Options

If you struggle with motivation, consider doing a "decisional balance exercise." When we think about making a change, most of us rarely consider all "sides" thoroughly. Instead, we often do what we think we "should" do, avoid doing things we don't feel like doing, or just feel confused or overwhelmed and give up thinking about it at all. Thinking through the pros and cons of both changing and not making a change is one way to help draw our motivation to the surface. It can also help us stay motivated in times of stress or temptation. Here's how it works. Using a chart like the one below, consider the SMART behavior you would like to add or change, and write all the pros and cons that come to mind regarding both making the change and not making the change.

	Pros	Cons
Making A Change		
Not Changing		

Once you consider your options, ask yourself which option seems the least painful in the long run? Which one could cause you the most regret if you didn't do it?

Make The Task Crystal Clear

When we set vague goals, such as "eat healthier" or "get to the gym at some point today," we're hoping that at some point in the future, a feeling of motivation will somehow come over us like a bolt of lightning. Unfortunately, this rarely happens.

To make it more likely that you'll take action, it's important to set clear, SMART goals, just as we discussed in Chapter 5. The clearer the goal, the more motivated you will feel to do it. Let's use meal prepping as an example. If you say that you'll try to meal prep at some point over the weekend, you'll likely keep putting it off until you have no choice but to say, "You know what, I have more important things to do. I'll just eat out this week."

Make meal prepping SMART:

Specific: *Here are the ingredients I will buy, the meals I will prepare, and the containers I will put them in.*

Measurable: *Here are portions and number of servings I need to prepare.*

Actionable: *Shopping, cooking, and portioning are all actions.*

Realistic: *Do you have the ability to cook, and do you have an hour or two to prepare the food?*

Timely: *Here's when I will shop, here's when I will start cooking, and here's how long it will take me to finish.*

Planning things out may spark the motivation to get up and get it done.

If exercising is your goal, have a very clear timeline of when you're going to do it. The difference between those who consistently exercise and those who don't is that those who exercise schedule what they're doing and when they're going to do it ahead of time. Instead of saying, "I'm going to the gym at some point tomorrow morning," commit to a specific time. "I'm going to wake up and change into my workout clothes so I can go to the gym right after breakfast."

Those who struggle wait to take action until they feel motivated, which doesn't happen. If you want to increase your motivation for a specific behavior, plan it out in advance. Don't wait. In this case the adage is correct: failing to plan is often planning to fail.

Be Careful With Visualization

One of the most common tips for getting motivated is to visualize success. While this sounds reasonable, research suggests that this might actually be counterproductive. People often visualize themselves achieving their goals but skip over visualizing all the effort that goes into making those goals a reality. By imagining that you have achieved your goal, you're actually depleting the amount of energy you have available to devote to accomplishing the task itself.

Alternatively, rather than imagining yourself having already succeeded, imagine all the necessary steps to get you there. What is the very next step? What challenges will you face? What strategies can you use to overcome those challenges? Anticipating the challenges you might encounter can make it easier to deal with them if they arise.

Should You Share Your Goals With Others?

Similar to visualization, a common belief is that sharing your goal with others will help you stay accountable. Unfortunately, this doesn't always happen, or if it does, it can have the opposite effect. People in your life who do try to hold you accountable may end up having the opposite effect and make you feel frustrated or discouraged.

In addition, sharing your goals with others can have another unforeseen side effect. Telling people what we're trying to do can change our social reality—it can feel like we have already achieved our goal, even though we haven't yet done the work. Telling someone our goal and having it acknowledged can feel good—so good, in fact, that our mind feels as if we've already succeeded. Because we've already felt the satisfaction, we're less likely to follow through with the consistent hard work that is necessary.

I know this sounds weird, but it is a real phenomenon introduced by the founder of social psychology, Kurt Lewin. It's called substitution.

Again, does this mean that you should never share your goals with others? Of course not! Everyone is different. What doesn't work for others might work for you. Research does suggest that, instead of telling people your end goal, you share with them what you're planning to do to achieve your goal. This way you focus more on the work instead of the outcome.

The Motivation Snowball

Many assume that we need to feel motivation before we take action. Oddly enough, motivation actually seems to get stronger after we start doing a certain behavior, not before. The strongest motivation develops as we actively engage in the process. As Newton's first law of physics states, objects in motion tend to stay in motion.

When doing a task, the greatest amount of friction lies right at the beginning. We feel it when we are sitting on the couch thinking about going to the gym or starting to meal prep. But once we are at the gym and are exercising, it takes less motivation to keep going. Once we've done the planning and the shopping and started cooking, meal prepping becomes easier to finish. Momentum carries us through, like a snowball effect. Let's look at how we can make getting started easier.

Shrinking The Task

According to Dr. BJ Fogg, a renowned behavior scientist at Stanford University, the amount of motivation necessary to complete a task is directly correlated with the difficulty of the task. The more daunting the task at hand, the more motivation is required to get started. However, if we shrink the task, making it smaller and more manageable, less motivation is needed to take action.

When a client of mine tells me they are having a hard time mustering up the motivation to take action on their weight-loss journey, it's often because they're trying to bite off more than they can chew. Big problems (or long journeys) are very rarely solved with big solutions. Instead, they are solved by a sequence of small solutions compounded over weeks, months, or longer. The hardest part lies in taking the first step.

Many report that the biggest challenge to working out is actually getting to the gym. Such was the case with a client of mine whom we'll call Nancy. After speaking to Nancy, we decided to implement a strate-

gy where we shrunk the task of working out at the gym: Nancy was going to plan out the days/times she was going to the gym, and on those
days, at first, all she had to do was walk into the gym and scan her card.
That's it!

For many, the best place to decide if you're going to work out is
when you're already at the gym. The worst place is sitting at home on
the couch. Once Nancy scanned her membership card at the front
desk, she would celebrate her success and go home. However, since she
was already at the gym, if she wanted to do some exercise once she
scanned her card, that was completely up to her. The only thing we
cared about was simply getting her to the gym.

Once she made a habit of getting to the gym, we then incrementally
increased the goal. Her next goal was to get to the gym and use the exercise bike for five minutes. Once that became consistent, we made it 10
minutes. Every few weeks, we gradually increased the duration. On any
given day, if she felt that the task was too daunting, she would lower the
expectation. For example, if her goal was 20 minutes but she felt too
tired and unmotivated to do it, she would say to herself, "At least get to
the gym and do five minutes. After that, if I still don't want to do it, I'll
leave." (Note: Nancy often did more than five minutes.)

Whenever I share this strategy with others, their knee-jerk reaction is
to roll their eyes and say, "This sounds like a waste of time. If you just
get to the gym and leave, or do only five to 10 minutes on the bike,
you're not really doing anything. What's the point?" Remember, each
journey starts with one single, tiny step. The point of this strategy is not
about how many Calories you're burning in the short-term; it's about
building consistency with exercise for the long-term. This is what taking

it one step at a time actually looks like. Focusing on this can pay you dividends in the long run.

This Isn't Supposed To Suck

We humans pursue activities that make us feel good and avoid those that make us feel bad. Many struggle to lose weight because they struggle with letting go of the belief that losing weight has to be miserable and uncomfortable in order to be effective. Take dieting, for example. If you google the word diet, you will see it defined as:

1. The kinds of food that a person, animal, or community habitually eats;

2. A special course of food to which one restricts oneself, either to lose weight or for medical reasons;

3. Restrict oneself to small amounts or special kinds of food in order to lose weight.

Two-thirds of that definition contain the word "restrict"! It's as if someone is saying to us, "Well, if you want to look good and be healthy, you have to give up everything that tastes good and provides you joy and comfort. Sorry."

It seems like we have to make a choice. Do we continue to be comfortable, eating what we enjoy, OR do we eat what will help us reach our goal? That's the problem. It's not an either-or scenario. It is absolutely possible to enjoy what you're eating and still achieve your results! In fact, that is how it should work. If you make changes that create a way of eating you cannot see yourself doing forever, it's wrong!

My clients who lost more than 20 pounds and kept it off all found ways of eating that met their Caloric goals AND that was enjoyable. That's how they stayed motivated to do it! Because they liked what they were eating and were getting results, they had no desire to stop.

If you're struggling with motivation around exercise or eating, perhaps the answer lies with finding things you do like. Resist the urge to restrict yourself, and instead, spend some time and energy researching healthy food options until you find some that you can see yourself eating long-term. Or try different types of physical activity until you find one you don't hate. This takes some investigating, but I assure you it is possible and very worthwhile.

The Biggest Mistake We Make About Motivation

While motivation can be a powerful force driving us to take action, waiting to feel motivated to take action is a mistake. While the strategies in this chapter will increase your motivation, they won't ensure that you will always be motivated because motivation is an inherently inconsistent feeling. Although motivation may be helpful in the beginning, it alone is not going to sustain our success. As world-record runner Jim Ryun said, "Motivation is what gets you started. Habit is what keeps you going." And that's what we're going to dive into next chapter—ways of breaking old habits and building new ones.

Key Points

- Motivation is the mental energy that makes us want to do something.

- Engaging in a decisional balance exercise can help you uncover and validate what you really want to do. It can also help you realize and plan for the difficulties.

- To increase motivation, make your tasks SMART. Sometimes a lack of motivation comes from a lack of clarity.

- Motivation increases with action, but getting started is often the hardest part.

- To get motivated to start a task, shrink the task until it becomes easy to do.

- Find ways to make the tasks enjoyable. If it feels like torture, it's a sign you're off track.

- At times, it is normal to feel unmotivated, which is why relying solely on motivation is not a good strategy for long-term success. Therefore, our focus should also be on building good habits.

Chapter 9

Habits

"Once you break a habit into its components, you can fiddle with the gears." -Charles Duhigg

E verything we are and everything we will achieve is a product of our habits. According to a study conducted at Duke University, around 40–45 percent of our daily behaviors are habits. While motivation is nice, our habits have the largest impact on our productivity, performance, and well-being. From our morning routine to our bedtime rituals and everything in between, habits make us who we are.

Therefore, it stands to reason that if we want to figure out our own path to success, we must understand the science and psychology behind what habits are and how they are formed. Doing so will enable you to build a stronger blueprint for cracking your code.

Why Habits?

As complex as our brains are, they have only a few main goals, one of which is energy conservation. Our brains are always looking for the path of least resistance. Habits enable us to be productive without expending much mental energy so that we can save it for other tasks. As a habit starts to form in our brain, it becomes more automatic, enabling our brain to work less and less. Eventually, our brain can virtually shut down and perform that task on autopilot.

Think about your drive to work. I bet that when you drove to your place of work for the first time (unless you were familiar with the area), you had no idea where you were going. You had to stay super alert to make sure you followed your GPS, didn't miss any turns, were in the correct lane, and were aware of your surroundings. Your brain used a lot of mental energy during that drive. However, as time went on, that drive got much easier. Now, not only do you no longer need your GPS, there are probably days when you completely zone out on your way to work because that drive is so automatic. Your brain uses far less mental energy now than it did when you first took that drive.

The whole point of habits is to conserve brainpower, which helps us function optimally and, ultimately, helps us survive. But to use habit formation in our favor, we first must understand how habits develop.

How Habits Are Formed

Habits form through repetition, but that's just part of the story. Habits exist in an area of the brain known as the basal ganglia. In his best-selling book, The Power of Habit (highly recommended), Charles Duhigg described something called the "habit loop" discovered by a group of MIT researchers. It is a sequential pattern that outlines how all habits are formed. Here's a snapshot:

Trigger causes a Behavior which gives us a Reward

When our brain engages in a rewarding behavior, our brain starts paying attention to that behavior. When we do it a few more times, our brain starts drawing a connection between the behavior and the reward. For example, if eating chocolate ice cream makes you happy, your brain starts to pay attention. If you do it more frequently in a short period of time, your brain starts connecting the ice cream with happiness.

Once that connection has been made, your brain needs a way to identify when the habit should occur, so it creates a trigger that causes it to switch into ice-cream-seeking mode. This trigger could be a place, a person, an object, a TV show, another behavior, or an emotion.

If we're feeling sad (trigger) and our brain is seeking out a way for us to be happy (reward), the behavior that our brain knows will work is eating chocolate ice cream. The more chocolate ice cream helps us go from sad to happy, if even for only a few moments, the stronger the habit becomes. Eventually, as soon as we feel sad enough, our brain goes into autopilot, and the next thing we know, we're eating chocolate ice cream (as long as it's easily available at the time... a factor we will discuss a little later).

Building A Good Habit

Once you understand how habits form, you can use this formula to build goal-producing habits into your life. Let's say you want to get into the habit of walking on the treadmill. The first step is to create a trigger for your habit. Research has shown the best way to do this is to pair the desired habit with a current habit, which is called habit stacking.

To create a habit of walking on the treadmill, the strategy would be to plan the desired behavior to occur immediately before or immediately after something you already do during the day. To get an idea of your options, create a list of things you typically do during the day, for example:

> You wake up.
> You go to the bathroom.
> You brush your teeth.
> You eat meals.
> You drive to work.
> You drive home from work.
> You arrive home from work.
> You take a shower.
> You go to bed.

As you look over your list, you might decide that the best time to walk on the treadmill is as soon as you arrive home from work. Once you make this decision, your goal is to arrive home, put on your workout clothes, and immediately jump on the treadmill. The more you do this sequence, the more of a habit it will become. This is just an example though; the key is to pick a sequence that will work for you.

Once you find a trigger that works, it's time to think about the reward section of the habit loop. Rewards are powerful because they typically satisfy an urge. However, identifying rewards can be challenging because we're not always aware of the urges that drive our behavior.

This is where improving our self-awareness and honing our investigative skills come in.

True, walking on a treadmill has many benefits, but for a reward to be effective, it needs to be immediate. One study showed that exercise adherence improved when the participants ate a piece of chocolate after their workout. On the surface, this may sound counterproductive, but for some it can be quite effective. Remember that you're the detective—find what works best for you.

Consider that the best reward usually comes from within. Many people say the best part of working out is the feeling they get after the workout. After you're done walking on the treadmill, focus on how you feel. Keep reminding yourself of how this behavior is benefiting you now and in the future. Let yourself experience the joy of accomplishment. As your brain connects walking with feeling great, it can become its own very powerful reward.

Changing Bad Habits

Now that we discussed the framework for building a new habit, let's discuss how to break habits that are less desirable. Technically, once a habit is stored in our basal ganglia, it cannot be erased, which means to be successful, we have to place a more productive habit on top of the current one. This is a lot easier read than done, but it is certainly doable.

The key to changing a habit once again lies with the habit loop. The problem is that, as with most other things, there is no one way to change a habit. Like everything else we've discussed in this book, you must use the formula in a way that works for you. To start, instead of creating a trigger and a reward like we did when building a habit, we need to do the opposite. We first must examine the habit we would like to change and reverse engineer it to uncover the current trigger and reward for the behavior.

Let's say you have a "bad" habit of eating about 400 Calories' worth of Doritos when you get home from work. Maybe you moved them from the counter to the top cabinet, thinking that it will make you less likely to eat them. You say that tomorrow you'll muster up the willpower to resist the Doritos, but tomorrow the habit takes hold again. How do you go about changing the behavior?

The first step is to become aware of the routine, which is pretty simple: it's the behavior you would like to change. In this case, it's eating Doritos when you arrive home from work.

The second step is more challenging. What's the reward? Is it the Doritos themselves? Is it satisfying hunger? Is it a way to pass the time until dinner? Is it relieving stress? Figuring this out will take some investigating.

Investigating different rewards is often helpful. On the first day of your investigation, when you get home and feel the urge, adjust your routine so that it delivers a different reward. For example, instead of grabbing the chips, grab a banana. The next day, as soon as you arrive home, go outside, walk around the block, and when you get back home, don't eat anything. The next day, grab a glass of water and sit in front of the TV.

It doesn't really matter what you choose to do instead of eating the Doritos. The point is to test different hypotheses to figure out which craving is driving your habit. If hunger is the craving, the banana should suffice. If it is boredom, watching TV might help. If it's stress or fatigue, walking around the block might make you feel better.

Once you've identified the reward, the next step is to identify the trigger for the routine. Remember, a trigger could be a location, a time, an emotional state, other people, or an immediately preceding action. Is your cue simply getting home from work? Is it when you look at your phone and see the time? Is it stress from the day? Stress from a phone call you got or didn't get? Fatigue? Boredom? Hunger? To identify your trigger, try answering the following questions the moment the craving strikes you:

Where are you?

Who else is around?

What time is it?

What's your emotional state?

What were you doing right before the craving hit?

When you identify both the trigger and the reward for a certain habit, you can begin to come up with a SMART plan for changing it. When triggered, plan to do something that will provide you with the same reward (i.e., will satisfy your hunger or will help you relax). Your new plan might sound something like this:

Every day, right when I get home from work, I will pour a glass of water, grab a banana from the basket, and sit down to watch TV for 30 minutes before cooking dinner.

Which Habit Should I Start Changing?

Making the necessary changes to successfully lose weight can feel overwhelming. The great news is that you don't have to change dozens of habits to be successful. You only have to change the few that will have a ripple effect on your outcomes.

Not all habits are created equal. Some habits are so powerful that they create a domino effect that leads to the development of multiple good habits. Habits like these are known as "keystone habits." An example of a keystone habit could be getting eight hours of sleep per night. Getting great sleep can create a ripple effect that leads to more positive outcomes, such as:

- more energy to work out

- improved decision-making ability

- decreased appetite due to normalization in hunger and satiety hormones (both of which are greatly affected by sleep)

- decreased stress levels

- enhanced mood

Consider making a list of all the habits you would like to develop or change, then pick one that you think might create a positive ripple effect in your life. Then use the information above for either building a new habit or changing an old one.

How Long Does Habit Change Take?

The popular belief is that it takes 21–30 days to create a habit. Unfortunately, this isn't true. It is an urban myth that all started with Dr. Maxwell Maltz, a plastic surgeon who performed rhinoplasty on his patients in the 1950s. Dr. Maltz found that after their nose job, it took his patients an average of 21 days to get used to their new face. He started incorporating his own life experiences into his theory, and in the 1960s published a book called Psycho-Cybernetics. Then, like the game telephone, this message seeped into society, spreading the belief that it takes 21–30 days to form a new habit.

Studies since have found that it takes an average of 66 days to form a habit. One study noted that it took anywhere from 18 to 254 days. How long it takes a new habit to form can vary widely depending on the behavior, the person, and the circumstances.

How Do I Stay Consistent Long Enough To Create A Habit?

Since it can take a while for a behavior to become a habit, what do we rely on to stay consistent? Is there something we can use after motivation fades and before a behavior becomes a habit? Indeed there is. It's called willpower, and it's the topic of our next chapter.

Key Points

- Habits are formed through a process known as the Habit Loop.

- For each habit there's a Trigger - the Habit itself - and a Reward.

- The first step in building a good habit, like going to the gym, is through Habit Stacking. This means pairing the behavior so that it takes place before or after an already established habit during the day.

- To change a bad habit, the key lies in reverse-engineering the habit loop. First, by finding the trigger and then replacing the bad habit with another, more beneficial behavior that still gives you the same reward.

- A powerful way to start is to find your Keystone habit(s).

- Contrary to popular belief, it can take much longer than 21-30 days to form a habit. Thus, we need to figure out a way to be good at self-control long enough for a behavior to become a habit.

Chapter 10

Willpower: The Bridge Between Motivation & Habits

"Willpower isn't something that gets handed out to some and not to others. It is a skill you can develop through understanding and practice." -Gillian Riley

Motivation gets us started and habits keep us going, but willpower is the bridge between the two. It is the ability to make good choices despite the temptations around us every day. In other words, willpower is the mental energy we use to resist doing something we crave doing. Figuring out how to remain in control of your choices, especially when you're not motivated, is paramount to achieving and maintaining your vision.

Although many view willpower as a form of mental toughness—being able to resist certain thoughts and wants—in 1994 a psychology professor at Harvard University named Daniel Wegner found that being in a constant state of resistance is almost always doomed to failure. Since then, many experts have agreed.

When we try to push away thoughts or cravings, such as "I want pizza," they can reemerge, often more intense than before, like a boomerang. Just like an insomniac who becomes more awake the harder they try to fall asleep, or a dieter who banishes carbs but can't stop thinking about them, the harder we try to resist an urge, the more likely we are to succumb to it. This concept is called ironic rebound.

So how do you overcome ironic rebound? By realizing the goal is not to resist and deprive ourselves. As simplistic as this seems, it is the answer. Yes, you want to allow yourself to enjoy your favorite foods from time to time, but more importantly, the key also lies with viewing willpower as a skill. To be consistent with goal-conducive behaviors is not about mental toughness; rather, it's about strategy and what you do to set yourself up for success.

Many people who struggle fall victim to the "willpower trap," or the assumption that if they are failing, it's because they haven't been blessed with good willpower. This simply isn't true. You can—and will—get better at mastering your willpower as long as you have the right mindset and strategies. In this chapter, we will discuss both: how to get good at the skill of making good decisions, whether you feel motivated or not; and the science behind willpower, as well as dozens of strategies that will help you avoid engaging in counterproductive behaviors.

Willpower 101

There are two main parts of our brain that determine our choices. Self-control comes from a part of our brain called the prefrontal cortex (PFC), which is the rational area of our brain that controls our decision-making. Impulses and emotions, on the other hand, come from our limbic system.

In the book Switch, authors Dan and Chip Heath share an analogy used by NYU psychologist Jonathan Hyde about how our brain interacts when it comes to decision-making and impulse control. Think of your brain like a rider on top of an elephant. The rider is the rational system, our prefrontal cortex. The elephant is our impulsive brain. Let's say the rider wants to go down a particular path, but the elephant doesn't because it's stressed, tired, or distracted. Who do you think will win?

This power imbalance is exactly what makes adopting new behaviors hard. The elephant always wins, even if the rational part of our brain, the rider, might want to go somewhere else. For this duo to move forward together on a journey, they need to agree, and they need to remove as many obstacles from their path as possible so that the elephant doesn't get spooked or frustrated and go out of control.

Ensuring The Rider Is Ready

Success is determined by us continuously making good choices that support our goals. In order for this to happen, the rider and the elephant need to stay in harmony with one another, and three crucial variables can affect this harmony: lack of sleep, increased stress, and unstable blood sugar. Let's take a look at each of them.

Sleep

The National Sleep Foundation recommends that we get seven to nine hours of sleep per night. While this sounds nice, it doesn't always happen. Whether it's because we work late, we want to watch another episode, or we stay out longer with friends, getting to bed earlier can be difficult. (And, as I'm finding out, if you have young children, getting enough sleep can sometimes feel downright impossible.)

Not only can sleep deficiency have health consequences such as hypertension, diabetes, and heart disease, it can also inhibit our weight-loss efforts. One study showed those who averaged less than seven hours of sleep per night gained twice as much weight as those who slept more than seven hours.

Sleep deprivation increases cortisol (which has been linked to increases in weight and body fat) and decreases our thyroid-stimulating hormone and growth hormone (our muscle tissue breaks down). It also increases the hunger-producing hormone ghrelin, while it decreases the satiety hormone leptin. In other words, a lack of sleep makes us hungrier more often, affects how long it takes us to feel full, and makes it more likely that we'll store body fat.

If that weren't bad enough, numerous studies have also shown that a lack of sleep impairs how the body and brain use glucose, one of our main energy sources. When we're tired, our cells have trouble absorbing glucose from the bloodstream, which makes our body and our brain desperate for energy. When we're desperate for energy, we start craving sweets and caffeine (fast energy sources). This is incredibly bad for self-control because it is one of the most energy-expensive tasks our brain can spend its fuel on.

Research has also demonstrated that when we are sleep deprived, we make decisions like we were mildly intoxicated. I don't know about you, but when I'm intoxicated, I don't make many good decisions.

Getting enough sleep could be a major keystone habit for a lot of us. Every night you get good rest makes a big difference. If you suspect sleep might be an issue for you, the first step is to determine if the issue is sleep quality or just the amount of time you spend in bed.

If it's the amount of time you're physically spending in bed, ask yourself what you are saying "yes" to instead of sleep. Is it snacking, watching TV, browsing social media, doing work? If this is something you might like to change, consider using the habit loop to build a habit of getting to bed earlier.

If you suspect sleep quality is the issue, the first step is to gain awareness regarding how much and how well you're currently sleeping. While you could go to the doctor for a sleep evaluation, the easiest way is to use a wearable device (e.g., Fitbit) that tracks your sleep patterns.

When it comes to being able to fall asleep, researchers believe that at least 50 percent of insomnia cases are stress related. Proven methods to purge stress before bed include deep-breathing exercises, meditation, exercising throughout the day, and keeping a gratitude journal.

If stress isn't the cause of your sleeping issue, consider developing a power-down ritual before bed. Since our bodies respond well to consistency, this starts by going to bed at the same time each night. Experts also suggest reading a book an hour before bed instead of using a laptop, tablet, TV, or phone. These devices contain blue light, which decreases the production of melatonin—also called the Dracula hormone, the hormone that helps us fall asleep. If giving up these devices is too much to ask, consider using blue-light-blocking glasses.

Other tips for improving sleep quality include setting the room temperature to between 66 and 72 degrees, making the room as dark as possible by shutting out or blocking any light, or using a white-noise machine. Remember, everything can work, but not everything will work for you. Investigate to find your own strategies for a better night's sleep.

Stress

According to the American Psychological Association, it is estimated that 75 percent of people suffer from stress, and stress plays a major role in weight gain for several reasons. One of the main ones deals with our hormones.

When we're stressed, our body releases a cascade of hormones, including adrenaline and cortisol, to create what's known as the fight-or-flight response. The release of adrenaline suppresses our appetite. However, as soon as the adrenaline wears off, we become ravenous. Our body shifts into a state where temptations become even more tempting and the part of our brain that controls willpower (our prefrontal cortex) becomes inhibited. This is why so many people habitually eat Calorie-dense foods (aka comfort foods) to ease stress.

If you have a health or fitness goal, reducing your stress levels may increase your chances of reaching your goal. While the causes and effects of stress in our lives can be complicated, if you feel stress is a major trigger for you, consider trying some of the scientifically proven strategies that follow.

We all depend on certain activities when stressed, including eating. The problem is that these activities are usually distractors, not relaxers. Distractors can also include shopping, smoking, drinking, binge-watching TV, and spending excessive amounts of time on social media. The reason these are ineffective methods of dealing with stress is that they release dopamine, a reward-seeking hormone. They make us feel like we're going to get a reward, but in the end we feel empty. In other words, we look forward to doing these things and they distract us, but ultimately, they don't make us feel any better.

If you want to stop relying on distractors, here are some strategies that have been proven to actually reduce stress:

- exercising/playing sports (as long as it's not too physically stressful)
- reading
- listening to your favorite music
- getting a massage
- going for a walk
- doing a creative hobby, such as coloring
- spending time with a pet (as long as they don't eat your furniture)
- deep-breathing exercises

One of the best strategies proven to both reduce stress AND increase self-control is meditation, which is like weight lifting for your brain. Meditation strengthens a number of self-control skills, including attention, focus, stress management, impulse control, and self-awareness. Meditation also increases blood flow to the PFC, and according to neuroscientists, it can rewire your brain. In fact, one study found eight weeks of daily meditation practice led to increased self-awareness and increased gray matter in areas of the brain related to stress and self-control. Meditation can become a solid keystone habit for many.

Blood Sugar

Have you ever heard the saying, "Never go grocery shopping when you're hungry"? The logic behind this is that when our blood sugar is low, we become impulsive. It's as if the elephant in our brain is starving and on a mission to eat.

Our brain has two main sources of fuel, oxygen and glucose. Glucose is measured in our body through blood sugar, and if it is too low, our brain turns us into a sugar-seeking monster. This is why we tend to crave carbs or sweets when our blood sugar gets low.

Not surprisingly, studies show that those who have normal blood-sugar levels are more likely to delay gratification. To keep your blood sugar normal and steady, consider avoiding highly processed, high-sugar foods, and eat foods with a low-glycemic index, such as lean proteins, beans, high-fiber grains, and many fruits and veggies. As always, observe your daily habits to see what strategies might be beneficial for you to investigate.

Decision Fatigue

Some have said that we make as many as 35,000 decisions each day, everything from what to wear to whether to go to the gym after work. One study asked people to guess how many food-related decisions they make in one day. The average guess was 14. The actual average number of food-related decisions was 227, many of which are subconscious!

This is important because the currency we use to make decisions is mental energy. Each time we make a decision, the less mental energy we have leftover. Throughout the day, we use our mental energy coping with fears, controlling spending, picking what to watch on TV, focusing on simple instructions, managing impressions of others, choosing what to eat, etc. As the day progresses, our mental energy bank gets closer and closer to zero. When our energy is depleted, we become a slave to our urges and impulses. This is called decision fatigue.

Too many people view themselves as lazy, when for many, what seems like laziness is often mental exhaustion. Change isn't hard because we are lazy or resistant; it's hard because we wear ourselves out! In other words, you aren't lazy; you might just be mentally, physically, and emotionally exhausted.

Therefore, if we want to consistently make better choices, we need to figure out ways to conserve and budget our mental energy. What follows is a menu of ideas that can help.

How To Set-up Your Environment For Success

We may think that we have full control over the choices we make, but a large number of our everyday actions are responses to our surroundings. The food in our pantry, the items on our desk at work, the over-abundance of addictive shows on Netflix—they all impact our behaviors in one way or another.

Our environment determines the default actions that we take on a day-to-day basis. Most of the time we don't consciously choose the environment that surrounds us; however, once we're aware of the effect it can have, we can take control and tweak it so that it works in our favor. As you start investigating how to change your behaviors, consider first making changes to your environment.

Remember this, if you're constantly surrounded by temptations, you will deplete your willpower trying to resist them, even subconsciously.

For instance, just knowing that your favorite Calorie-dense foods are in the house will slowly wear away at your willpower until you finally cave and eat them. One of the big keys to redesigning your environment is eliminating as many temptations as possible!

Imagine your world—your home, your office, etc.—being crafted in such a way that it made good behaviors easier and bad behaviors harder. How much more often would you make healthy, productive choices if they were simply your default response to your environmental triggers? How much easier would it make things if you weren't surrounded by as many temptations?

Designing your environment in such a way as to make the right behaviors more convenient and the wrong behaviors less convenient is called choice architecture. Here are a few examples that can give you some ideas that will help you redesign your own environment.

Out Of Sight, Out Of Mind

The easiest strategy to set up your environment so that you eat less is the "out of sight, out of mind" rule. Basically, if it's not in your house, you won't eat it. For example, if there are chips in my house, at some point during the day, I will make way to them and devour the entire bag. If they're not at home, though, I won't eat a single one.

Removing food can be challenging if you have a significant other or kids who demand that certain "bad" foods be kept in the house. If this is your reality, try finding a strategy that makes that food less visible to you. For example, tuck the cookies away in places you can't see or get to, and instead, place the more nutrient-dense foods in more visible spots in your refrigerator, pantry, and around the kitchen.

I've had clients who found it helpful to have others keep their "bad food" in a food safe to which my client didn't know the combination. Others find it helpful to have an open conversation with their loved ones, asking them not to eat that type of food in front of them. Explore whatever you think might work for you.

Shrink Your Dinnerware

Researchers have found that using smaller plates is a simple strategy for cutting Calories. In one experiment, it was discovered that a shift from 12-inch plates to 10-inch plates resulted in a 22 percent decrease in Caloric intake. Smaller plates cause us to eat less, thanks to a powerful optical illusion known as the Delboeuf illusion, illustrated below:

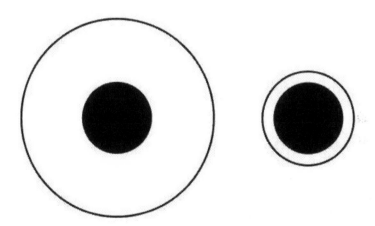

In the picture above, which black circle looks larger, the one on the left or the one on the right? Most will say the one on the right but in reality, they're exactly the same size! This is a prime example of the Delboeuf illusion.

If you put a small piece of food on a large plate, your mind will tell you that you are eating a small portion and you will automatically put more food on your plate. However, if you put that same amount of food on a small plate, your mind will tell you that you are eating a larger portion and you'll stop adding food. Try storing your dinner plates in the closet, and eat dinner on your salad plates. You may find that it helps.

Remember, the goal when changing your environment is to make good behaviors easier and to put obstacles in the way of bad behaviors. To lower your liquid Calorie intake, try using smaller glasses. It will force you to physically get up from the table (obstacle) to keep refilling (as long as you keep the soda in the refrigerator instead of on the table). Conversely, if you want to drink more water, do the exact opposite. Drink from larger vessels, such as a 32-ounce water bottle, and if you use a water pitcher during dinner, keep it on the table to make it easier to drink more water.

Other Examples Of Choice Architecture

There are so many ways you can alter your environment for positive change. If you want to avoid that fast-food restaurant you pass on the way home, consider taking an alternative route.

If you want to work out in the morning, try laying out your workout clothes the night before or even sleeping in them. When the morning comes, there will be one less barrier in your way.

Having trouble getting out of bed in the morning? Try putting your alarm clock (or phone) across the room, forcing you to get out of bed to shut it off.

This works for goals other than changing your eating or exercising. Let's say your goal is to read more and watch less television. You could put the remote in a drawer, closet, or somewhere else out of sight and place a good book where the remote used to be. This increases the likelihood that you'll pick up the book and start reading.

The more inconvenient you make the bad choices, the less frequently you'll make them. The more convenient you make the good choices, the more likely you WILL make them. What are some ways you could make your environment more conducive to success?

Getting The Right Support

It's not just our physical environment that affects our choices; our social environment can play an even larger role. We are all shaped by the people around us. Finding the right amount of support can be the difference between failure and success.

When it comes to the people in our lives and their impact on our choices, we can usually separate them into two categories: friends and accomplices. Friends are those who support our goals and help us achieve them. Maybe they model the right behaviors, have the right attitude, or provide us with the encouragement we need to be successful. We just seem to do better in their presence.

And then there are the accomplices. They are our partners in crime —the ones who talk us out of exercising, talk us into ordering that extra appetizer or dessert, and make being unhealthy seem normal. While in their presence, we find ourselves in an environment full of temptations, apathy, and peer pressure.

Thinking of your loved ones in this way may sound a little harsh. But the truth is, the people who surround us (at home and socially) really do make achieving our goals either easier or harder.

Here's an example. Let's imagine you're dining out at a restaurant with a group of people. If everyone at the table orders wine, an appetizer, a salad, an entrée, and a dessert, you're likely going to do the same. Saying no to any of the above would make you the odd one at the table, and nobody wants to feel like that.

However, if you're at the table with friends who are more health-conscious, drink only water, and order only an entree, you will be less likely to order an appetizer or dessert because, again, that would make you the weird one.

Please understand that I'm not implying that if someone is an "accomplice" you need to stop seeing them. It may just mean that you need to spend more time with good influences to shift the social scale in the right direction.

Here are some ways you can do this:

- Get a workout partner or partners.

- Attend support groups where you'll be surrounded by people who will encourage you. Weight watchers is a popular example, but there are many others. If you don't like any in your area, you can also create one of your own (e.g., start a neighborhood walking club).

- Hire a personal trainer, nutritionist, and/or health coach to help you on your journey.

- Speak with your spouse or a good friend about accompanying you on this journey toward health and fitness. This could be an example of turning an "accomplice" into a "friend."

- Join an Internet community.

- The more time you spend with those who will help you achieve your goals, the better you will do and the less affected you'll be by the accomplices in your life.

Skillpower > Willpower

Willpower is not about learning how to resist temptations; instead, it's about figuring out ways to avoid them or to distract yourself from them. The first step is understanding your triggers/temptations as discussed in the last chapter. Next, you need to investigate and experiment with different tweaks to your physical and/or social environment until you find what works for you.

Willpower is a skill you absolutely can master! Once you figure out the strategies that work for you, there is no limit on what you can achieve.

Key Points

- Willpower is the mental energy used to take action toward a goal, especially when it requires you to resist your urges. It is the same thing as self-control.

- Many believe in the self-limiting myth that self-control is a natural talent that some have and others don't. In actuality, self-control is a skill that it based more on strategy than inner strength.

- Quality sleep, stable blood sugar and lower levels of stress are necessary for your brain to be in the ideal state for willpower.

- Willpower is an exhaustible resource. The more we need to resist our urges and make decisions, the lower our capacity for self-control becomes.

- Setting up our environment for success will make good decisions easier and bad decisions harder. It will also reduce the need to resist urges, thus saving our mental energy.

- Social support is also a big key to success for most. The more friends you have instead of accomplices, the more help you'll have to crack your code.

- Willpower, like anything else we've discussed in this book is about understanding and developing new skills.

Conclusion

"Nothing will work unless you do." -Maya Angelou

Anyone who tells you that losing weight is easy is either completely out of their mind or trying to sell you something. Literally thousands of experts and companies will claim to have cracked the code to losing weight. They will try to get you to buy their step-by-step programs and to follow their advice—often with a patronizing tone.

The fact is, the formula for weight loss was discovered a long time ago. If your energy expenditure exceeds your energy intake, you will lose weight. This is not a mystery, despite what some may tell you. As we've discussed throughout this book, the true mystery lies in figuring out what unique combination of methods and strategies will enable you to adhere to this formula with your schedule and priorities.

Which habits do you need to change? How will you go about changing them? What or who will help support you in your efforts? What obstacles do you encounter? What strategies will help you work around these obstacles? These are the questions you need to dig into and figure out.

Doing this successfully starts with your mindset, which is predicated on two central beliefs. The first is the belief that, to be successful, you need to take control of your own journey. Nobody is going to give you all the answers and do this for you. This is your mystery to solve, your code to crack! If you want your goals to become a reality, you must willingly take on the role and responsibilities of being the lead detective. This means having an unwavering commitment to continue the iterative process of trial and learning until you arrive at your answers.

The second belief is that you are capable of being successful. I know that YOU CAN DO THIS. The question is, do you believe that you can? There will always be marketers and experts trying to make you feel broken, trying to convince you there's an easier way and that you should "invest" in their step-by-step system. They profit from you having the "passenger mindset." Please remember that everybody struggles, despite what the airbrushed world of social media might lead you to believe. Your failures are not proof of hopelessness; they're clues to get you closer to your goal.

Throughout this book, we discussed a process for cracking your code and finding a solution to whatever obstacle you're encountering—whether it's nutrition, not being motivated to exercise, willpower, or building good habits. This processed can be summarized with the following chart:

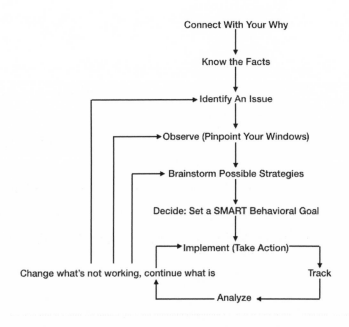

Having a "detective's mindset" means always keeping an open mind and believing that the answer is out there somewhere—you just have to keep digging deeper. Instead of throwing in the towel, keep asking yourself, "What am I overlooking?" With constant curiosity and guided experimentation, you will find the answers you're searching for!

This Is A Journey, Not A Destination

While we have reached the end of this book, we have also reached the beginning of a brand-new journey for you. You're not embarking on this journey for the reasons society tells you that you should; you're doing it for the reasons you feel are important—to achieve your vision.

As you go about cracking your code, think of this book as a resource to refer to whenever the need arises, especially since this journey to a thinner, healthier, happier you never really concludes, it merely evolves. From time to time, new obstacles and setbacks will arise. Perhaps your schedule will change, or you will have a baby, or you will move. No matter where you are on your journey, there will always be new strategies to try and new skills to learn.

Nobody Ever Learned To Swim By Reading

Reading a book like this will provide you with concepts and principles to help you be successful. However, reading by itself will not get you where you want to be. You must work to apply the principles by taking action, even if you don't feel ready.

When working on a big journey toward something important, it is normal to feel like you need more time to "think it over" or prepare. You will feel unprepared and uncertain, but this is when the best discoveries are made! Don't let this deter you from getting started. After all, you can't begin the process of trial and learning if you don't first try.

Final Thoughts

It's time to embrace the fact that there has never been nor will there ever be another person in this universe like you! Everything about you and your journey is what makes you unique! Your system for losing weight should reflect your unique needs, preferences, DNA, obstacles, and lifestyle. Right now it's a mystery, but hopefully this book has given you some insight about how to find your path to a thinner, healthier and happier life.

On a journey like this, it's easy to temporarily lose your way and want to give up. Please remember that there are always tweaks you can make and possible strategies to investigate. Don't be afraid of failure—it's a wonderful teacher. Each day, week, and month has the potential to reveal a crucial piece of the puzzle. Your code is out there somewhere!

All change starts with the first small step. Small steps become big steps. Big steps become leaps until you find yourself living your vision. Once this happens, you will have done what many struggle to do—you will have cracked your code. Happy investigating!

– Chris

P.S. Let me know how you're doing along the way. Have a question? Don't hesitate to reach out to me. Send me an email (chris@chrisbarlic-s.com). I'd love to hear from you! You can also find me on Facebook and Instagram.

Bonus Resources

THANK YOU so much for taking the time to read this book. I hope you found it helpful. If you are looking of more tools and resources to help you on your journey, then allow me to make a suggestion.

Since you read this book, you have exclusive access to the free, reader's only bonuses I've created. To find out what they are, simply go to:

chrisbarlics.com/crack-your-code-resources

Notes

Chapter 1

Foxcroft, L. How We Fought Fat Throughout History. Retrieved from https://www.bbc.com/timelines/z9nfyrd

Office on Smoking and Health (US). Women and Smoking: A Report of the Surgeon General. Atlanta (GA): Centers for Disease Control and Prevention (US); 2001 Mar. Chapter 4. Factors Influencing Tobacco Use Among Women.

Fujioka, K., Greenway, F., Sheard, J., et al. 2006. The effects of grapefruit on weight and insulin resistance: relationship to the metabolic syndrome. J. Med Food; 9:49-54.

Wikipedia contributors. (2019). WW International. In Wikipedia, The Free Encyclopedia. Retrieved 01:07, July 4, 2019, from https://en.wikipedia.org/w/index.php?title=WW_International&oldid=905096485

Catherine Zeratsky. (2006, May 4). What Is the Cabbage Soup Diet? Retrieved from https://www.mayoclinic.org/healthy-lifestyle/weight-loss/expert-answers/cabbage-soup-diet/faq-20058079

Ann F. La Berge. 2008. How the Ideology of Low Fat Conquered America. Journal of the History of Medicine and Allied Sciences. 63(2), 139–177. https://doi.org/10.1093/jhmas/jrn001

Police, S. 2013. How Much Have Obesity Rates Risen Since 1950? Retrieved from https://www.livestrong.com/article/384722-how-much-have-obesity-rates-risen-since-1950/

Crescent, B.M., Herrick, K.A., Sarafrazi, N., and Cynthia L Ogden. 2018. Attempts to Lose Weight Among Adults in the United States, 2013-2016. NCHS Data Brief. No.313. Retrieved from https://www.niddk.nih.gov/health-information/health-statistics/overweight-obesity

The U.S. Weight Loss & Diet Control Market. Feb 2019. Market Data LLC. Retrieved from https://www.researchandmarkets.com/research/qm2gts/the_72_billion?w=4

National Weight Control Registry. Research Findings. Retrieved from http://www.nwcr.ws/research/

Chapter 2

Pash, C. (2013, Nov 22). Meet The Australian Personal Trainer Who Showed The World Before And After Photos Are Pointless. Retrieved from
https://www.businessinsider.com.au/meet-the-australian-personal-trainer-who-showed-the-world-before-and-after-photos-are-pointless-2013-11

McGonigal, Kelly. 2012. The Willpower Instinct: How Self-control Works, Why It Matters, and What You Can Do to Get More of It. New York: Avery.

Çetin, B , Gündüz, H , Akın, A . (2016). An Investigation Of The Relationships Between Self-Compassion, Motivation, And Burnout With Structural Equation Modeling[English]. Abant İzzet Baysal Üniversitesi Eğitim Fakültesi Dergisi, 8 (2), . Retrieved from http://dergipark.org.tr/aibuefd/issue/1495/18082

Trumpeter, N., P.J. Watson and B.J. O'Leary. 2006. "Factors within Multidimensional Perfectionism Scales: Complexity of Relarips with Self-Esteem, Narcissism, Self-Control, and Self-Criticism." Personality and Individual Differences 41: 849-860.

Chapter 3

Moore, Margaret, Jackson, E., Tschannen-Moran, Bob & Wellcoaches Corporation (2015). Coaching psychology manual 2nd edition. Lippincott, Williams & Wilkins, Philadelphia.

Cleveland Clinic. Obesity is top cause of preventable life-years lost, study shows." ScienceDaily. ScienceDaily, 22 April 2017. <www.sciencedaily.com/releases/2017/04/170422101614.htm

Chapter 4

Hill, J. O., Wyatt, H. R., & Peters, J. C. (2012). Energy balance and obesity. Circulation, 126(1), 126–132. doi:10.1161/CIRCULATIONAHA.111.087213

Hill, J. O., Wyatt, H. R., & Peters, J. C. (2013). The Importance of Energy Balance. European endocrinology, 9(2), 111–115. doi:10.17925/EE.2013.09.02.111

Hafekost, K., Lawrence, D., Mitrou, F., O'Sullivan, T. A., & Zubrick, S. R. (2013). Tackling overweight and obesity: does the public health message match the science?. BMC medicine, 11, 41. doi:10.1186/1741-7015-11-41

Strasser B., Spreitzer A., Haber P. Fat loss depends on energy deficit only, independently of the method for weight loss. Ann. Nutr. Metabol. 2007;51:428–432. doi: 10.1159/000111162.

Wikipedia contributors. 2019. Calorie. In Wikipedia, The Free Encyclopedia. Retrieved from https://en.wikipedia.org/w/index.php? title=Calorie&oldid=906447895

J. Berardi and R. Andrews. The Essentials of Sport and Exercise Nutrition. 2013. Precision Nutrition.

Frankenfield D, Roth-Yousey L, Compher C. Comparison of predictive equations for resting metabolic rate in healthy nonobese and obese adults: a systematic review. J Am Diet Assoc. 2005;105:775–789.

A new predictive equation for resting energy expenditure in healthy individuals. Mifflin MD, St Jeor ST, Hill LA, Scott BJ, Daugherty SA, Koh YO. Am J Clin Nutr. 1990 Feb; 51(2):241-7.

McArdle W (2006). Essentials of exercise physiology. Lippincott Williams & Wilkins. p. 266.

J. Berardi and R. Andrews. The Essentials of Sport and Exercise Nutrition. 2013. Precision Nutrition.

McCall, P. (2017, Nov 21). 6 Things to Know About Non-exercise Activity Thermogenesis. Retrieved from https://www.acefitness.org/education-and-resources/lifestyle/blog/6852/6-things-to-know-about-non-exercise-activity-thermogenesis

Kelly, M. (October 2012). Resting Metabolic Rate: Best Ways to Measure It - and Raise It, Too. Retrieved from https://www.acefitness.org/certifiednewsarticle/2882/resting-metabolic-rate-best-ways-to-measure-it-and/

Wishnofsky M. Caloric equivalents of gained or lost weight. Am J Clin Nutr. 1958;6:542–546.

Ferdman, R.A. (2015, July 28). Why the Most Popular Rule of Weight Loss Is Completely Wrong. Retrieved from https://www.washingtonpost.com/news/wonk/wp/2015/07/28/why-the-most-popular-rule-of-weight-loss-is-completely-wrong/?utm_term=.2495f5522eb1

A third of UK adults 'underestimate calorie intake.' 2018, Feb 19. Retrieved from https://www.bbc.com/news/health-43112790

St. Pierre, B. 2019. The Best Calorie-Control Guide. Retrieved from https://www.precisionnu-trition.com/calorie-control-guide-infographic

Mawer, R. (2016, June 14). Calorie Cycling 101: A Beginner's Guide. Retrieved from https://www.healthline.com/nutrition/calorie-cycling-101#section6

Schwartz A, Doucet É. Relative changes in resting energy expenditure during weight loss: a systematic review. Obes Rev 2010; 11: 531–547.

American College of Sports Medicine,, Riebe, D., Ehrman, J. K., Liguori, G., & Magal, M. 2018. ACSM's guidelines for exercise testing and prescription (Tenth edition.). Philadelphia: Wolters Kluwer.

Chapter 5

Kaufman, J. 2010. The Personal MBA : A world-class business education in a single volume New York : Portfolio Penguin.

TEDx Talks. "Change anything! Use skill power over willpower| Al Switzler| TEDxFremont." Filmed [Noc 2012]. YouTube video, 19:02. Posted [Dec 2012]. https://www.youtube.com/watch?v=3TX-Nu5wTS8

Frey, M. 2019, March 29. Is Weight Fluctuation Normal? How Much Daily Weight Fluctuation You Should Expect. Retrieved from https://www.verywellfit.com/why-does-weight-change-day-to-day-4100012

Stoddard, G. 2018, Oct 29. This Is What Happens to Your Body if You Eat Almost No Carbs. Retrieved from https://www.vice.com/en_us/article/negxgw/this-is-what-happens-to-your-body-if-you-eat-almost-no-carbs

Chapter 6

Stelmach-Mardas, M., Rodacki, T., Dobrowolska-Iwanek, J., Brzozowska, A., Walkowiak, J., Wojtanowska-Krosniak, A., … Boeing, H. 2016. Link between Food Energy Density and Body Weight Changes in Obese Adults. Nutrients, 8(4), 229. doi:10.3390/nu8040229

George Washington University. 2019. Children and teens who drink low-calorie sweetened beverages do not save calories: New study also shows kids and teens who consume low-calorie sweetened beverages take in more calories compared to those who drink water. ScienceDaily. Retrieved July 1, 2019 from www.sciencedaily.com/releases/2019/05/190502075832.htm

Jr., C. R. (2017, July 18). Diet drinks are associated with weight gain, new research suggests. Retrieved from https://www.washingtonpost.com/news/to-your-health/wp/2017/07/18/diet-drinks-are-associated-with-weight-gain-new-research-suggests/?utm_term=.c2bb62f66025

Get the Facts: Drinking Water and Intake | Nutrition | CDC. 2016. Retrieved from https://www.cdc.gov/nutrition/data-statistics/plain-water-the-healthier-choice.html

Corney R.A., Sunderland C., James L.J. 2016. Immediate pre-meal water ingestion decreases voluntary food intake in lean young males. Eur. J. Nutr. 55:815–819. doi: 10.1007/s00394-015-0903-4.

Jeong J. N. 2018. Effect of Pre-meal Water Consumption on Energy Intake and Satiety in Non-obese Young Adults. Clinical nutrition research, 7(4), 291–296. doi:10.7762/cnr.2018.7.4.291

Boschmann M, Steiniger J, Hille U, Tank J, Adams F, Sharma AM, Klaus S, Luft FC, Jordan J. Water-induced thermogenesis. J Clin Endocrinol Metab. 2003;88:6015–6019.

Yoquinto, L. (2011, June 24). 25% of Calories Now Come from Snacks. Retrieved from https://www.livescience.com/14769-snacking-calories-increase.html

Wu, Helen, Sturm, & Roland. (2012, January 01). Some Menus of U.S. Sit-down Chain Restaurants Are as Unhealthy as Fast Food. Retrieved from https://www.rand.org/pubs/external_publications/EP201200113.html#related

Chandler-Laney, P. C., Morrison, S. A., Goree, L. L., Ellis, A. C., Casazza, K., Desmond, R., & Gower, B. A. 2014. Return of hunger following a relatively high carbohydrate breakfast is associated with earlier recorded glucose peak and nadir. Appetite, 80, 236–241. doi:10.1016/j.appet.2014.04.031

Myers, D. (2017, December 11). Why Do Restaurants Give You Bread? Retrieved from https://www.thedailymeal.com/eat/why-do-restaurants-give-you-bread

McGonigal, K. (2012). The willpower instinct: How self-control works, why it matters, and what you can do to get more of it. New York, NY, US: Avery/Penguin Group USA

Maruyama, K., Sato, S., Ohira, T., Maeda, K., Noda, H., Kubota, Y., ... Iso, H. 2008. The joint impact on being overweight of self reported behaviours of eating quickly and eating until full: cross sectional survey. BMJ (Clinical research ed.), 337, a2002. doi:10.1136/bmj.a2002

Ohkuma T, Hirakawa Y, Nakamura U, et al. 2015. Association between eating rate and obesity: a systematic review and meta-analysis. Int J Obes (Lond), 39:1589–96.

Leong SL, Gray A, Horwath CC. 2016. Speed of eating and 3-year BMI change: a nationwide prospective study of mid-age women. Public Health Nutr; 19:463–9

Kokkinos A., le Roux C.W., Alexiadou K., Tentolouris N., Vincent R.P., Kyriaki D., Perrea D., Ghatei M.A., Bloom S.R., Katsilambros N. 2010. Eating Slowly Increases the Postprandial

Response of the Anorexigenic Gut Hormones, Peptide YY and Glucagon-Like Peptide-1. J. Clin. Endocrinol. Metab.; 95:333–337. doi: 10.1210/jc.2009-1018.

Neal, D. T., Wood, W., Wu, M., & Kurlander, D. (2011). The Pull of the Past: When Do Habits Persist Despite Conflict With Motives? Personality and Social Psychology Bulletin, 37(11), 1428–1437. https://doi.org/10.1177/0146167211419863

Chapter 7

DeRose, S. (2017, September 14). Rutgers Football, Eric LeGrand and One Simple Word: Believe. Retrieved from https://bleacherreport.com/articles/566247-rutgers-football-eric-legrand-and-one-simple-word-believe

Ussery, E. N., Fulton, J. E., Galuska, D. A., Katzmarzyk, P. T., & Carlson, S. A. 2018. Joint Prevalence of Sitting Time and Leisure-Time Physical Activity Among US Adults, 2015-2016. JAMA, 320(19), 2036–2038. doi:10.1001/jama.2018.17797

HHS Office, & Council on Sports. (2017, January 26). Facts & Statistics. Retrieved from https://www.hhs.gov/fitness/resource-center/facts-and-statistics/index.html

Jaslow, R. (2013, May 03). CDC: 80 percent of American adults don't get recommended exercise. Retrieved from https://www.cbsnews.com/news/cdc-80-percent-of-american-adults-dont-get-recommended-exercise/

Cimons, M. (2017, August 12). Exercise does so much for you. Why won't it make you lose weight? Retrieved from https://www.washingtonpost.com/national/health-science/exercise-does-so-much-for-you-why-wont-it-make-you-lose-weight/2017/08/11/618db370-77d7-11e7-8f39-eeb7d3a2d304_story.html?utm_term=.8d5e52e4c12a

Belluz, J., & Haubursin, C. (2019, January 02). The science is in: Exercise won't help you lose much weight. Retrieved from https://www.vox.com/2018/1/3/16845438/exercise-weight-loss-myth-burn-calories

A. Luke, R. S. Cooper. 2014. Physical activity does not influence obesity risk: time to clarify the public health message. International Journal of Epidemiology. 42 (6): 1831 DOI: 10.1093/ije/dyt159

Harvard Health Publishing. (n.d.). Calories burned in 30 minutes for people of three different weights. Retrieved from https://www.health.harvard.edu/diet-and-weight-loss/calories-burned-in-30-minutes-of-leisure-and-routine-activities

American College of Sports Medicine, Deborah Riebe, Jonathan K. Ehrman, Gary Liguori, and Meir Magal. 2018. ACSM's guidelines for exercise testing and prescription.

Cheung K., Hume P. A., Maxwelf L. 2003. Delayed Onset Muscle Soreness: Treatment strategies and performance factors. Sport Med. 33 145–164. 10.2165/00007256-200333020-00005

Robinson, J. (n.d.). Overtraining: 9 Signs of Overtraining to Look Out For. Retrieved from https://www.acefitness.org/education-and-resources/lifestyle/blog/6466/overtraining-9-signs-of-overtraining-to-look-out-for

10 Signs You're Exercising Too Much. (n.d.). Retrieved from https://health.usnews.com/health-news/blogs/on-fitness/2010/11/05/10-signs-youre-exercising-too-much

Dellitt, J. (2019, June 21). Overexercising: What It Means and How to Know When to Stop. Retrieved from https://aaptiv.com/magazine/overexercising

Digest, R. (2017, December 14). Exercising too much can actually make you gain weight - here's why. Retrieved from https://www.businessinsider.com/exercising-too-much-can-actually-make-you-gain-weight-heres-why-2017-12

Fry, R. W., Grove, J. R., Morton, A. R., Zeroni, P. M., Gaudieri, S., & Keast, D. (1994). Psychological and immunological correlates of acute overtraining. British journal of sports medicine, 28(4), 241–246. doi:10.1136/bjsm.28.4.241

4 rules for avoiding overuse injuries. (2019, January 08). Retrieved from https://www.mayoclinic.org/healthy-lifestyle/fitness/in-depth/overuse-injury/art-20045875

Metabolism. (2019, July 20). Retrieved from https://en.wikipedia.org/wiki/Metabolism

Fothergill, E., Guo, J., Howard, L., Kerns, J. C., Knuth, N. D., Brychta, R., Chen, K. Y., Skarulis, M. C., Walter, M., Walter, P. J., and Hall, K. D.. " Persistent Metabolic Adaptation 6 Years after 'The Biggest Loser' Competition." Obesity, 24, 2016, 1612– 19. https://doi.org/10.1002/oby.21538.

Deering, K. 2015. How to Heal Your Metabolism: Learn How the Right Foods, Sleep, the Right Amount of Exercise, and Happiness Can Increase Your Metabolic Rate and Help Heal Your Broken Metabolism. Createspace.

Steen, J., & Steen, J. (2017, January 19). This Is Why Detoxes (Really) Don't Work. Retrieved from https://www.huffingtonpost.com.au/2017/01/18/so-detoxes-or-cleanses-dont-work-heres-why_a_21657800/

Lee S, Kim M, Lim W, Kim T, Kang C. Strenuous exercise induces mitochondrial damage in skeletal muscle of old mice. Biochem Biophys Res Commun. 2015;461(2):354–60.

Feito, Y., Heinrich, K. M., Butcher, S. J., & Poston, W. 2018. High-Intensity Functional Training (HIFT): Definition and Research Implications for Improved Fitness. Sports (Basel, Switzerland), 6(3), 76. doi:10.3390/sports6030076

Harvard Health Publishing. (n.d.). The truth about metabolism. Retrieved from https://www.health.harvard.edu/staying-healthy/the-truth-about-metabolism

McCall,P. (n.d.). 4 Myths about Strength Training for Women. Retrieved from https://www.acefitness.org/education-and-resources/professional/expert-articles/5040/4-myths-about-strength-training-for-women

Deering, K. 2015. How to Heal Your Metabolism: Learn How the Right Foods, Sleep, the Right Amount of Exercise, and Happiness Can Increase Your Metabolic Rate and Help Heal Your Broken Metabolism. Createspace.

J. Berardi and R. Andrews. The Essentials of Sport and Exercise Nutrition. 2013. Precision Nutrition.

Chapter 8

Pressfield, Steven. 2012. The War of Art: Break through the blocks and win your inner creative battles. New York : Black Irish Entertainment

Heath, Chip and Dan Heath. 2010. Switch: how to change things when change is hard. New York: Broadway Books.

Kappes, H. B., & Oettingen, G. 2011. Positive fantasies about idealized futures sap energy. Journal of Experimental Social Psychology, 47(4), 719-729. https://doi.org/10.1016/j.jesp.2011.02.003

Gollwitzer, P. M., Sheeran, P., Michalski, V., & Seifert, A. E. 2009. When Intentions Go Public: Does Social Reality Widen the Intention-Behavior Gap? Psychological Science, 20(5), 612–618. https://doi.org/10.1111/j.1467-9280.2009.02336.x

James Clear. (n.d.). Motivation: The Scientific Guide on How to Get and Stay Motivated. Retrieved from https://jamesclear.com/motivation

James Clear. (2018, July 13). I'm Using These 3 Simple Steps to Actually Stick with Good Habits. Retrieved from https://jamesclear.com/small-habits

Chapter 9

Neal, D. T., Wood, W., & Quinn, J. M. 2006. Habits—A Repeat Performance. Current Directions in Psychological Science, 15(4), 198–202. https://doi.org/10.1111/j.1467-8721.2006.00435.x

Clear, James. 2018. Atomic Habits: An Easy & Proven Way to Build Good Habits & Break Bad Ones. New York: Avery, an imprint of Penguin Random House.

Duhigg, Charles. 2012. The Power of Habit : Why We Do What We Do in Life and Business. New York : Random House.

Clear, James. 2018. Atomic Habits: An Easy & Proven Way to Build Good Habits & Break Bad Ones. New York: Avery, an imprint of Penguin Random House.

Duhigg, Charles. 2012. The Power of Habit : Why We Do What We Do in Life and Business. New York : Random House.

Seger, C. A., & Spiering, B. J. 2011. A critical review of habit learning and the Basal Ganglia. Frontiers in systems neuroscience, 5, 66. doi:10.3389/fnsys.2011.00066

Duhigg, Charles. 2012. The Power of Habit : Why We Do What We Do in Life and Business. New York : Random House.

James Clear. (2018, July 13). How Long Does it Take to Form a Habit? Backed by Science. Retrieved from https://jamesclear.com/new-habit

Lally,P., van Jaarsveld, C.H.M., Potts, H.W.W., and J. Wardle. 2010. How are habits formed: Modelling habit formation in the real world. European Journal of Social Psychology. 6: 40: 998-1009

Chapter 10

Wegner, D.M. 1994. Whte Bears and Other Unwanted Thoughts: Suppressions, Obesession, and the Psychology of Mental Control. New York: Guilford Press.

Wegner, Daniel M. 2009. How to think, say, or do precisely the worst thing for any occasion. Science 325(5936): 48-50.
Published Version

Richard M. Wenzlaff and Daniel M. Wegner. 2000. Thought Suppression. Annual Review of Psychology 51:1, 59-91

Giuliano, R.J., and N.Y. Wicha. 2010. "Why the White Bear is Still There : Electrophysiological Evidence for Ironic Semantic Activation During Thought Suppression." Brain Research 1316: 62-74

Patterson, K., Granny, J;, Maxfield, D, McMillan, R., and Al Switzler. 2011. Chang Anything: The New Science of Personal Success. New York: Business Plus.

Coutlee, C. G., & Huettel, S. A. (2012). The functional neuroanatomy of decision making: prefrontal control of thought and action. Brain research, 1428, 3–12. doi:10.1016/j.brainres.2011.05.053

Heath, Chip, and Dan Heath. 2010. Switch: how to change things when change is hard. New York: Broadway Books.
National Sleep Foundation Recommends New Sleep Times. (n.d.). Retrieved from https://www.sleepfoundation.org/press-release/national-sleep-foundation-recommends-new-sleep-times

Leproult, R., & Van Cauter, E. (2010). Role of sleep and sleep loss in hormonal release and metabolism. Endocrine development, 17, 11–21. doi:10.1159/000262524

Patel SR, Malhotra A, White DP, Gottlieb DJ, Hu FB. Association between reduced sleep and weight gain in women. Am J Epidemiol. 2006; 164:947-54.

Beccuti, G., & Pannain, S. (2011). Sleep and obesity. Current opinion in clinical nutrition and metabolic care, 14(4), 402–412. doi:10.1097/MCO.0b013e3283479109

Xiao, Q., Arem, H., Moore, S. C., Hollenbeck, A. R., & Matthews, C. E. 2013. A large prospective investigation of sleep duration, weight change, and obesity in the NIH-AARP Diet and Health Study cohort. American journal of epidemiology, 178(11), 1600–1610. doi:10.1093/aje/kwt180

Spiegel, K., Tasali, E., Leproult, R., & Van Cauter, E. 2009. Effects of poor and short sleep on glucose metabolism and obesity risk. Nature reviews. Endocrinology, 5(5), 253–261. doi:10.1038/nrendo.2009.23

Killgore W.D.S., Kahn-Greene E.T., Lipizzi E.L., Newman R.A., Kamimori G.H., and T.J. Balkin. 2008. Sleep deprivation reduces perceived emotional intelligence and constructive thinking skills. Sleep Medicine. 9:517–526.

Kalmbach, D. A., Pillai, V., & Drake, C. L. 2018. Nocturnal insomnia symptoms and stress-induced cognitive intrusions in risk for depression: A 2-year prospective study. PloS one, 13(2), e0192088. doi:10.1371/journal.pone.0192088

The Best Ways to Relieve Stress and Tension So You Can Sleep Soundly. (n.d.). Retrieved from https://www.sleepfoundation.org/articles/learn-leave-stress-behind-bedtime

This Is the Best Temperature for Sleeping, According to Experts. (n.d.). Retrieved from https://www.health.com/sleep/best-temperature-for-sleeping

Best Temperature for Sleep. (n.d.). Retrieved from https://www.sleep.org/articles/temperature-for-sleep/

Basaraba, S. (2019, July 22). How the Soothing Tones of White Noise Can Help You Sleep Better. Retrieved from https://www.verywellhealth.com/white-noise-and-sound-sleep-2224280

American Psychological Association. 2010. Stress in America. 1-64: Washington, DC.
Sapolsky, R. M. 1994. Why zebras don't get ulcers: A guide to stress, stress related diseases, and coping. New York: W.H. Freeman.

American Psychological Association. 2007. Stress in America. Washington, DC.

Anton, B.S. 2016. Coping with Stress. Monitor on Psychology Vol 46, (11), p5.

J. A. Brefczynski-Lewis, A. Lutz, H. S. Schaefer, D. B. Levinson, R. J. Davidson. 2007. Neural Correlates of Attentional Expertise in Long-term Meditation Practitioners. Proceedings of the National Academy of Sciences 104: 11483-11488.

Hölzel, B. K., Carmody, J., Vangel, M., Congleton, C., Yerramsetti, S. M., Gard, T., & Lazar, S. W. 2011. Mindfulness practice leads to increases in regional brain gray matter density. Psychiatry research, 191(1), 36–43. doi:10.1016/j.pscychresns.2010.08.006

Wang, X.T., and R.D. Dvorak. 2010. Sweet future: fluctuating blood glucose levels affect future discounting. Psychological Science 21: 183-188.

Wansink, B., & Sobal, J. 2007. Mindless Eating: The 200 Daily Food Decisions We Overlook. Environment and Behavior, 39(1), 106–123. https://doi.org/10.1177/0013916506295573

Baumeister, Roy F., and John Tierney. 2012. Willpower: rediscovering the greatest human strength. New York: Penguin Books.

Baumeister, R.F., T.F. Heatherton, and D.M. Time. 1994. Losing Control: How and Why People Fail at Self-Regulation. San Diego: Academic Press.

Thaler, R.H., and C.R. Sunstein. 2008. Nudge: Improving Decisions About Health, Wealth, and Happiness. New York: Knopf.

Thorndike, A. N., Sonnenberg, L., Riis, J., Barraclough, S., & Levy, D. E. 2012. A 2-phase labeling and choice architecture intervention to improve healthy food and beverage choices. American journal of public health, 102(3), 527–533. doi:10.2105/AJPH.2011.300391
McClain, A. D., van den Bos, W., Matheson, D., Desai, M., McClure, S. M., & Robinson, T. N. 2014. Visual illusions and plate design: the effects of plate rim widths and rim coloring on perceived food portion size. International journal of obesity (2005), 38(5), 657–662. doi:10.1038/ijo.2013.169

Sharp, D., & Sobal, J. 2012. Using plate mapping to examine sensitivity to plate size in food portions and meal composition among college students. Appetite, 59(3), 639–645. doi:10.1016/j.appet.2012.07.020 Note: The Validity of plate size related to portion control has been called into question within the last few years. This strategy may work for some, but not for others. For more information see also...Zitron-Emanuel, N., Ganel, R. 2018. Food deprivation reduces the susceptibility of size-contrast illusions. Appetite. 128:138-144.

Rothgerber, H. (2015). Can you have your meat and eat it too? Conscientious omnivores, vegetarians, and adherence to diet. Appetite, 84, 196-203. doi:10.1016/j.appet.2014.10.012

Christakis, N.A., and J.H. Fowler. 2007. The Spread of Obesity in a Large Social Network over 32 years. New England Journal of Medicine 357: 370-379.

Carrell, S.E., M.Hoekstra, and J. E. West. 2010. Is Poor Fitness Contagious? Evidence and Randomly Assigned Friends. Working Paper 16518, National Bureau of Economic Research.

Powell, K., Wilcox, J., Clonan, A., Bissell, P., Preston, L., Peacock, M., & Holdsworth, M. 2015. The role of social networks in the development of overweight and obesity among adults: a scoping review. BMC public health, 15, 996. doi:10.1186/s12889-015-2314-0

Patterson, K., Granny, J;, Maxfield, D, McMillan, R., and Al Switzler. 2011. Chang Anything: The New Science of Personal Success. New York: Business Plus.

Index

Made in the USA
Middletown, DE
13 September 2020